CT & MRI PATHOLOGY

A Pocket Atlas

Third Edition

T0175969

Michael L. Grey, PhD, RT(R), (CT)(MR), FASRT
Professor, Emeritus
Radiologic Sciences
MRI/CT Specialization
Southern Illinois University

Jagan M. Ailinani, MD
Medical Director, Imaging Department (Retired)
Memorial Hospital of Carbondale
Clinical Professor of Radiology and Community Medicine
(Retired)
Southern Illinois University School of Medicine, Springfield,
Illinois

Mc
Graw
Hill
Education

New York   Chicago   San Francisco   Athens   London   Madrid
Mexico City   Milan   New Delhi   Singapore   Sydney   Toronto

CT & MRI: Pathology: A Pocket Atlas, Third Edition

3 4 5 6 7 8 9 LCR 23 22 21

ISBN 978-1-260-12194-0
MHID 1-260-12194-1

NOTICE

Medicine is an ever-changing science. As new research and clinical experience broaden our knowledge, changes in treatment and drug therapy are required. The authors and the publisher of this work have checked with sources believed to be reliable in their efforts to provide information that is complete and generally in accord with the standards accepted at the time of publication. However, in view of the possibility of human error or changes in medical sciences, neither the authors nor the publisher nor any other party who has been involved in the preparation or publication of this work warrants that the information contained herein is in every respect accurate or complete, and they disclaim all responsibility for any errors or omissions or for the results obtained from use of the information contained in this work. Readers are encouraged to confirm the information contained herein with other sources. For example and in particular, readers are advised to check the product information sheet included in the package of each drug they plan to administer to be certain that the information contained in this work is accurate and that changes have not been made in the recommended dose or in the contraindications for administration. This recommendation is of particular importance in connection with new or infrequently used drugs.

This book was set in Adobe Jenson Pro by MPS Limited.
The editors were Susan Barnes and Cindy Yoo.
The production supervisor was Catherine Saggese.
Project management was provided by Vivek Khandelwal at MPS Limited.
The designer was Mary McKeon.

This book is printed on acid-free paper.

Library of Congress Cataloging-in-Publication Data

Names: Grey, Michael L., author. | Ailinani, Jagan M., author.
Title: CT & MRI pathology : a pocket atlas / Michael L. Grey, Jagan M. Ailinani.
Other titles: CT and MRI pathology
Description: Third edition. | New York : McGraw-Hill Education, [2018]
Identifiers: LCCN 2018008718| ISBN 9781260121940 (pbk. : alk. paper) | ISBN 1260121941 (pbk. : alk. paper)
Subjects: | MESH: Tomography, X-Ray Computed—methods | Magnetic Resonance Imaging—methods | Atlases | Handbooks
Classification: LCC RC78.7.T6 | NLM WN 17 | DDC 616.07/5722—dc23
LC record available at https://lccn.loc.gov/2018008718

McGraw-Hill Education books are available at special quantity discounts to use as premiums and sales promotions or for use in corporate training programs. To contact a representative, please visit the Contact Us pages at www.mhprofessional.com.

CONTENTS

CONTRIBUTING AUTHORS

Michael Erik Landman, MD
Department of Radiology
Vanderbilt University Medical Center

Neal Weston Langdon, MD
Department of Radiology
Vanderbilt University Medical Center

Kim L. Sandler, MD
Department of Radiology
Vanderbilt University Medical Center

PREFACE

In this third edition of the *CT and MRI Pathology: A Pocket* Atlas, several new additions have been included. Probably the first noticeable new addition is the section titled *CT and MRI Contrast Agents*. This section contains an overview of the pertinent issues concerning contrast agents used in CT and MRI. New cases in cardiac, spine, a series of hernia cases, and additional musculoskeletal cases have been added throughout the book to increase the breadth of this new edition.

ACKNOWLEDGMENTS

I would like to express my gratitude to my wife Rebecca and my children Kayla, Emily, and Megan for allowing me time away from home to complete this new edition. Many thanks to all the wonderful people around the United States and throughout the world who have benefited from this book and their kind compliments.

It has been 30 years since my initial diagnosis of cancer. I would like to thank my Lord and Savior Jesus Christ for His loving grace and mercy, and the many miracles I have seen and experienced along life's journey.

Thank you,
Michael

First, I am grateful to all of you who made the first edition of the *CT & MRI Pathology: A Pocket Atlas* so popular in 2003 that it led to the second edition in 2012 and now to the third edition. I would like to thank Michael Grey for all his support and help. Finally, I would like to thank my wonderful wife Uma for always being there for me.

Thank you,
Jagan

SPECIAL ACKNOWLEDGMENTS

From the initial publication of the first edition of CT & MRI Pathology: A Pocket Atlas textbook in 2003 to this current third edition many individuals have given me invaluable support and encouragement and helped to see this book through. To them I have thanked and given credit in previous editions.

Along life's journey, others have come and influenced my life in special ways, and I would like to take this opportunity to express my deep appreciation to them. Without these people, I know that I would not be where I am today.

Charles Coffey II

Jackie Darling

Ho See Kim

Steve and Cathy Jensen

Paul Mills

Marilyn Paulk

Paul Sarvela

I am forever grateful to God for these friends and how they have touched my life.

Thank you all!

Michael L. Grey

NUCLEAR MAGNETIC RESONANCE IMAGING (NMRI)

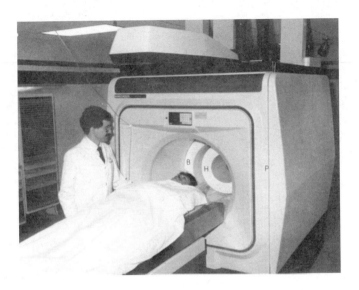

This is a photo of the first commercially made Nuclear Magnetic Resonance (NMR) Imaging unit in the world. NMR Imaging is commonly referred to today as Magnetic Resonance Imaging (MRI).

This photo shows the Head coil (H), the Body coil (B) in the center of the bore, and the plastic housing (P). This NMR unit was a Technicare 0.15T Resistive system. As a show site to the world, visitors were frequent, and many tours were given to introduce this new technology to the world.

This photo was taken in the mid-1980s. By that time, several companies had also begun producing their own NMR units. The gentlemen posing for this photo are Michael Grey (standing) and the service engineer (positioned on the patient couch).

PART I

Principles of Imaging in Computed Tomography and Magnetic Resonance Imaging

PRINCIPLES OF IMAGING IN COMPUTED TOMOGRAPHY AND MAGNETIC RESONANCE IMAGING

Since the initial discovery of x-ray by Wilhelm Conrad Roentgen on November 8, 1895, the field of radiology has experienced two major breakthroughs that have revolutionized how we look into the patient's body. The first, computed tomography (CT) came in the early 1970s. The second, magnetic resonance imaging (MRI) was initially introduced in the early 1980s.

In CT, a finely collimated x-ray beam is directed upon the patient. As the x-ray tube travels around the patient, x-rays are emitted toward the patient. As these x-rays interact with the various tissues in the patient's body, some of the x-rays are attenuated by the tissues while others are transmitted through the tissues and interact with a very sensitive electronic detector. The purpose of these detectors is to measure the amount of radiation that has been transmitted through the patient. After the amount of radiation has been measured, the detector converts the amount of radiation received into an electronic signal that is sent to a computer. The computer then performs mathematical calculations on the information received and reconstructs the desired image. This information is assigned a numerical value that represents the average density of the tissue in that respective pixel/voxel of tissue. These numerical values reflect the patient's tissue attenuation characteristics and may be referred to as Hounsfield numbers, Hounsfield units (HU), or CT numbers that range from approximately -1000 (air) to $+3000$ (dense bone or tooth enamel). CT uses water as its standard value and it is assigned a Hounsfield number of 0.

To diagnose a disease process, the radiologist looks for changes in the normal density (HU) of an organ, an abnormal mass, or an altered or loss of normal anatomy. The advantages of CT include its ability to image patients that (1) have experienced trauma, (2) are suspect to have had a stroke, (3) are acutely ill, (4) have a contraindication to MRI, or (5) require better bone detail that can be scanned in CT in a quick and efficient manner. In addition, since the development of helical (spiral) CT in the early 1990s with single-slice technology and further technological advances in the mid-1990s to multi-slice imaging, CT is able to perform volumetric imaging quickly and generate reformatted anatomic images in any plane (e.g., sagittal or coronal). The disadvantages of CT include (1) exposure to the radiation dosage, (2) possible reaction to the iodinated contrast agent, (3) lack of direct multiplanar imaging, and (4) loss of soft-tissue contrast when compared to MRI.

MRI incorporates the use of a strong magnetic field and smaller gradient magnetic fields in conjunction with a radiofrequency (RF) signal and RF coils specifically tuned to the Larmor frequency of the proton being imaged. An image is acquired in MRI by placing the patient into a strong magnetic field and applying an RF signal at the Larmor frequency of the hydrogen proton (42.58 MHz/T). Gradient magnetic fields are used to assist with spatial localization of the RF signal. The gradients are assigned to the tasks of slice selection, phase encoding, and frequency encoding or readout gradient. In the magnet, the patient's hydrogen protons align either parallel (with) or antiparallel (against) the magnetic field. The RF signal is rapidly turned on and off. When the RF signal is turned on, the protons are flipped away from the parallel axis of the magnetic field. Once the RF is turned off, the protons begin to relax back into the parallel orientation of the magnetic field. During the relaxation time, a signal from the patient is being received by the coils and sent to the computer for image reconstruction. This process is repeated several times until the image is acquired.

There are several different types of pulse sequences used in MRI to acquire patient information. These can be grouped into proton (spin) density, and T1-weighted and T2-weighted pulse sequences. These pulse sequences demonstrate the anatomy differently and help differentiate between normal and abnormal structures. A combination of these pulse sequences may be used to assist with the diagnosis.

A T1-weighted pulse sequence uses a short TR (repetition time) and short TE (echo time) values to produce a high or bright signal in substances such as fat, acute hemorrhage, and slow-flowing blood. Structures such as cerebrospinal fluid and simple cysts may appear with a low or dark signal. In many cases, the pathologic process will appear with low signal in T1-weighted images.

A proton-density-weighted image uses long TR and short TE values to produce images based on the concentration of hydrogen protons in the tissue. The brighter the area, the greater the concentration of hydrogen protons. The darker the area, the fewer the number of hydrogen protons.

A T2-weighted pulse sequence uses long TR and long TE values to obtain a high signal in substances such as cerebrospinal fluid, simple cysts, edema, and tumors. Structures such as fat and muscle will appear with low signal. Many pathologic conditions present with high signal on T2-weighted pulse sequences.

MRI has several advantages such as (1) it acquires patient information without the use of ionizing radiation; (2) it produces excellent soft tissue contrast; (3) it can acquire images in the transverse (axial), sagittal, coronal, or oblique (orthogonal) planes; and (4) image quality is not affected by bone. The disadvantages primarily associated with MRI would include: (1) any contraindication that would present a detrimental effect to the patient or health care personnel; (2) long scan time when compared to CT; and (3) cost. The effects of the magnetic field, varying gradient magnetic fields, or the RF energy used pose the greatest harmful effects to biomedical implants that may be in the patient's body. Before entrance into the strong magnetic field can be obtained, everyone including patients, family members, health care professionals, and maintenance workers must be screened for any contraindications that may result in injury to themselves or others. These may include any biomedical implant or device that is electrically, magnetically, or mechanically activated such as pacemakers, cochlear implants, and certain types of intracranial aneurysm clips and orbital metallic foreign bodies. The contraindications focus on devices that may move or undergo a torque-effect in the magnetic field, overheat, produce an artifact on the image, or become damaged or functionally altered. Most magnets used in MRI are superconductive and the magnetic field is always on. Any ferromagnetic material (e.g., O_2 tank, wheelchairs, stretchers, scissors) may become a projectile and potentially cause an injury or death when brought into the magnetic environment.

PART II

Contrast Media

CT AND MRI CONTRAST AGENTS

Technologists working in computed tomography (CT) or magnetic resonance imaging (MRI) are responsible for performing a wide variety of examinations on a diverse population of patients. Many of these examinations require the use of a contrast agent. It is very important, therefore, that the technologist has a working knowledge of how to perform venipuncture and how to safely administer the specific contrast agent required. To safely administer a contrast agent, the technologist must be able to determine five things:

- The specific contrast agent to be used;
- The correct amount to be used;
- The appropriate injection site;
- The correct injection rate; and
- The appropriate gauge of the IV needle to be used.

Upon the completion of the examination, all pertinent details of the venipuncture and administration of the contrast agent should be documented in the patient chart by the technologist, along with the overall patient outcome. To ensure the safety of the patient, it would be beneficial for the technologist to have an overview of the main points to consider prior to using either a CT or an MRI contrast agent.

CT Contrast Agents

Water-soluble contrast agents, which consist of molecules containing atoms of iodine, are used extensively in CT. Although risk of adverse reaction is low, there is a real risk inherent in their use which can run from mild to life threatening. Due to these safety risks, newer but more expensive, low-osmolar contrast agents have replaced the older, cheaper high-osmolar ionic contrast agents. Adverse side effects are uncommon for these agents ranging from 5% to 12% with ionic to 1% to 3% with nonionic, low-osmolality intravascular contrast agents.

Mild reactions are the most common type of reaction and usually do not require treatment. Patients experiencing any of the typical reactions should be observed for 30 minutes following the onset to ensure that the reaction does not become more severe. Common signs and symptoms include:

- Nausea/vomiting.
- Urticaria/pruritis.

- Sneezing.
- Itchy/scratchy throat.
- Feeling warm/chills.
- Headache/dizziness/anxiety/altered taste.

Moderate reactions are not life threatening but commonly require treatment for symptoms. Some of these reactions may become severe if not treated. Common signs and symptoms include:

- Diffuse urticaria/pruritis.
- Diffuse erythema, stable vital signs.
- Facial edema without dyspnea.
- Throat tightness or hoarseness without dyspnea.
- Wheezing/bronchospasm, mild or no hypoxia.
- Protracted nausea/vomiting.
- Isolated chest pain.
- Vasovagal reaction that requires and is responsive to treatment.

Patients should be monitored until symptoms resolve. Benadryl is effective for relief of symptomatic hives. Beta agonist inhalers help with bronchospasm (wheezing) and epinephrine is indicated for laryngeal spasm. Leg elevation (Trendelenburg position) is indicated for vasovagal reaction and hypotension.

Severe reactions, which are potentially life-threating reactions, usually occur within the first 20 minutes following the intravascular injection of contrast. Severe reactions are rare but should be recognized and treated immediately. Common signs and symptoms include:

- Diffuse edema, or facial edema with dyspnea.
- Diffuse erythema with hypotension.
- Laryngeal edema with stridor and/or hypoxia.
- Anaphylactic shock (hypotension with tachycardia).
- Vasovagal reaction resistant to treatment.
- Arrhythmia.
- Convulsions, seizures.
- Hypertensive emergency.

Severe bronchospasm or severe laryngeal edema may progress to unconsciousness, seizures, hypotension, dysrhythmias, cardiac arrest, and needs immediate cardiopulmonary resuscitation.

Local side effects, such as extravasation of the contrast agent at the injection site, may cause pain, swelling, skin slough, and deeper tissue necrosis. The affected limb should be elevated. Warm compress may help with absorption of the contrast agent while a cold compress is more effective in reducing pain at the injection site. With the current use of power injectors, extra care should be taken in observing the injection site during the administration phase of the contrast agent.

While the terms extravasation and infiltration have been used interchangeably, a difference should be noted. An infiltration is the inadvertent administration of a non-vesicant fluid (i.e., normal saline) into the surrounding tissues. An extravasation is the inadvertent administration of a vesicant fluid (i.e., contrast agent, chemotherapy) into the surrounding tissue. A vesicant fluid can cause necrosis or tissue damage when it escapes from the vein.

Contrast-Induced Nephropathy

Contrast-induced nephropathy (CIN) is defined as acute renal failure (sudden deterioration in renal function) occurring within 48 hours of contrast injection and is a significant source of morbidity. CIN is a subgroup of post-contrast acute kidney injury (AKI). Most prominent risk factors are diabetes and chronic renal insufficiency. Adequate hydration is essential in the prevention of CIN. Patients should be encouraged to drink several liters of water/fluid 12 to 24 hours before and after intravascular administration of contrast. As a prophylactic treatment, an intravenous bolus of N-acetylcysteine (Mucovit) may also be recommended at a dose given orally (600 mg twice daily) on the day before, and on the day of contrast administration. Another option is that 500 ml of normal saline is given over 30 minutes prior to the exam and 500 ml of normal saline over 4 hours after the examination.

Metformin (Glucophage)

Metformin (Glucophage) is an oral antihyperglycemic agent used to treat type 2 diabetes mellitus. It may potentially cause fatal lactic acidosis. Metformin should be discontinued for 48 hours following an iodinated contrast administration and reinstated only after renal function is reevaluated and found to be normal.

High-risk patients for adverse contrast reactions should be identified and consideration given as to whether a contrast agent should be given. In cases where administrating a contrast agent may not be in the best interest of the patient, alternative imaging such as ultrasound may be helpful. Further, it may be possible for the radiologist to monitor the non-contrast CT exam to assess the images as they are acquired. If contrast is needed, the patient should be adequately hydrated. Premedication should be considered.

Risk factors include the following:

1. Previous history of adverse reaction to intravenous contrast.
2. Clear history of asthma or allergies. A history of an allergy to shellfish or iodine is not a reliable indicator of a possible contrast reaction.

3. Known cardiac dysfunction including severe congestive heart failure, severe arrhythmias, unstable angina, recent myocardial infarction or pulmonary hypertension.
4. Renal insufficiency, especially in patients with diabetes mellitus.
5. Sickle cell disease.
6. Multiple myeloma.
7. Age over 65.

All the patients having CT contrast should be screened appropriately. For patients at risk for reduced renal function, serum creatinine/eGFR (glomerular filtration rate) is to be obtained. Technologists need the patient's age, gender, weight, and serum creatinine to use the GFR calculator (found online). Patients who have a GFR of less than 30 ml/min, should not be given contrast.

Premedication has been proven to decrease but not eliminate the frequency of contrast reactions. Two regimens listed by American College of Radiology (ACR) include either:

1. Prednisone 50 mg taken orally at 13 hours, 7 hours, and 1 hour before contrast administration.
2. Methylprednisolone 32 mg taken orally at 12 hours and 2 hours prior to contrast administration.

Benadryl 50 mg orally, IM, or IV should be taken or given 1 hour prior to contrast for either of regimen (above).

Nonionic low-osmolality contrast should be used with either regimen (above).

MR Contrast Agents

Gadolinium chelates are the most commonly used MR contrast agents. These agents differ according to being either ionic or nonionic, and according to their osmolality and viscosity. Their distribution and elimination is very similar to water-soluble iodine-based contrast agents used in CT. Injected intravenously gadolinium chelates diffuse rapidly into extracellular fluid and blood pool spaces and are excreted by glomerular filtration. About 80% of an injected dose is excreted within 3 hours. MR imaging is usually done immediately after injection.

Adverse reactions to gadolinium contrast agents are quite uncommon. Common signs and symptoms for mild reactions include:

- Nausea/vomiting.
- Headache.
- Warmth or coldness at the injection site.

- Paresthesia.
- Dizziness.
- Itching.

Life-threatening reactions are rare. Gadolinium has no nephron toxicity at doses used for MR. Since gadolinium agents are radiopaque, they have been used in conventional angiography in patients with renal impairment or severe reaction to iodinated contrast.

Nephrogenic Systemic Fibrosis

Nephrogenic systemic fibrosis (NSF), originally described in 2000, is a systemic disorder characterized by widespread tissue fibrosis following the administration of a gadolinium-based contrast agent in individuals with noticeable advanced renal failure. This disease causes fibrosis of the skin and connective tissues throughout the body. Patients affected develop skin thickening that may prevent bending and extending of joints, resulting in their decreased mobility. Affected patients experience fibrosis that has spread to other parts of the body such as the diaphragm, muscles of the thigh and lower abdomen, and interior areas of the lung vessels. The clinical course is progressive and fatal.

High-risk patients for reduced renal function include:

- Age 65 or over.
- Diabetes mellitus.
- History of renal disease or renal transplants.
- History of liver transplantation, hepatorenal syndrome.

As a safety precaution, serum creatinine (eGFR) should be obtained in all patients with reduced renal function. Patients, who have a GFR of less than 30 ml/min, should not be given contrast.

Intravenous (IV) Contrast and the Pregnant Patient

The safety of fetal exposure to CT and MR contrast agents are not well described in the literature. The current recommendation is to avoid routine administration of contrast agents in pregnant patients unless the information is critical to the management of the patient (risk versus benefit). Alternate imaging studies like ultrasound also must be considered.

PART III

Central Nervous System

BRAIN
NEOPLASM

Acoustic Neuroma

Description: An acoustic neuroma, also known as a vestibular schwannoma, is a benign fibrous tumor that arises from the Schwann cells covering the vestibule portion of the eighth cranial nerve. These tumors are well encapsulated, compress but do not invade the nerve. Acoustic neuromas account for approximately 80% to 85% of all cerebellopontine angle (CPA) tumors and make up 10% of all intracranial tumors.

Etiology: There is no known cause for this tumor. Bilateral eighth cranial nerve schwannomas are pathognomonic for neurofibromatosis type II.

Epidemiology: Acoustic neuromas account for approximately 5% to 10% of all intracranial tumors. They are the most common tumors affecting the cerebellopontine angle. Males and females are affected equally. The average age of onset is between 40 and 60 years.

Signs and Symptoms: Sensorineural hearing loss, tinnitus, and vertigo are common in patients.

Imaging Characteristics: Note: MRI is the imaging modality of choice.

CT
- Well-rounded hypodense to isodense mass on noncontrast study.
- Hyperdense with contrast enhancement.

MRI
- T1-weighted (T1W) imaging without contrast is usually isointense to slightly hypointense.
- T1-weighted pulse sequence with contrast enhancement demonstrates the tumor with a marked enhancement.
- T2-weighted images may demonstrate an increase (hyperintense) in signal.
- Baseline imaging following surgery should include a precontrast T1-weighted and fat-suppression postcontrast pulse sequences.

Differential Diagnosis: Include mainly meningioma, metastasis, and paraganglioma.

Treatment: Surgery intervention is required.

Prognosis: Depending on the size of the acoustic neuroma, the prognosis is encouraging and usually is curative.

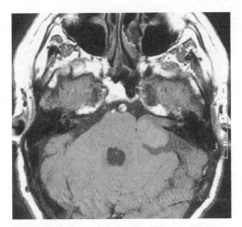

FIGURE 1. Acoustic Neuroma. Noncontrast T1-weighted axial image demonstrating round isointense mass at the left cerebellopontine (CP) angle.

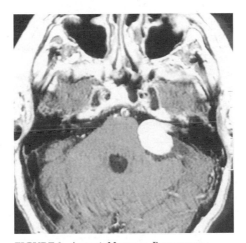

FIGURE 2. Acoustic Neuroma. Postcontrast T1-weighted axial image demonstrating an intense contrast enhancing extraaxial mass at the left cerebellopontine angle close to the left internal auditory canal (IAC) consistent with an acoustic neuroma.

Astrocytoma

Description: Astrocytomas are the most common primary intracranial neoplasm. They originate from the astrocysts of the brain. The World Health Organization (WHO) subdivided astrocytomas into four histologic grades: Grade I (circumscribed astrocytoma); Grade II (diffuse astrocytoma); Grade III (anaplastic astrocytoma); and Grade IV (glioblastoma multiforme).

Etiology: Unknown.

Epidemiology: Account for approximately 10% to 30% of cerebral gliomas in adults.

Signs and Symptoms: Typically are associated with an increase in pressure within the skull. May include headaches, visual problems, change in mental status, seizures, and vomiting.

Imaging Characteristics: Approximately two-thirds of all low-grade astrocytomas are located above the tentorium (supratentorial), mainly in the frontal, temporal, and parietal lobes of the cerebrum.

CT
- Helpful when MRI is contraindicated.
- Appear as poorly defined, homogeneous, hypodense mass without IV contrast.
- Enhances with IV contrast; however, cyst does not enhance.
- Calcification seen in less than 10%.
- Edema and mass effect may be seen.

MRI
- T1-weighted images appear hypointense.
- T2-weighted images appear hyperintense.
- T1-weighted with IV contrast shows enhancement.
- Fluid attenuated inversion recovery (FLAIR) images show hyperintense tumor.
- Edema and mass effect may be seen.

Treatment: Surgery and radiation therapy.

Prognosis: When detected early and removed completely, a good prognosis (5-year survival rate >90%) is possible.

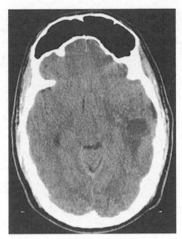

FIGURE 1. **Astrocytoma.** Axial
NECT of the head shows a low-
attenuation mass in the left temporal
lobe with surrounding edema.

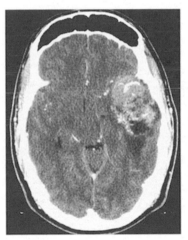

FIGURE 2. **Astrocytoma.** Axial CECT
shows mild enhancement of the mass
which contains areas of necrosis.

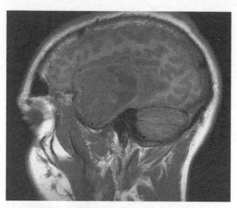

FIGURE 3. **Astrocytoma.** Sagittal T1W image shows an isointense mass in the left temporal lobe with surrounding low signal edema.

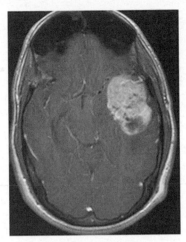

FIGURE 4. Astrocytoma. Postcontrast axial T1W image shows enhancement of the mass in the left temporal lobe. There is mass effect on the surrounding brain with effacement of the left ambient cistern.

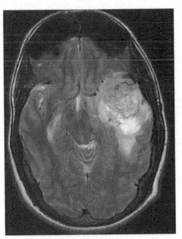

FIGURE 5. Astrocytoma. Axial T2W image shows the left temporal mass with surrounding high-signal edema.

Brain Metastasis

Description: Brain metastasis is the metastatic spread of cancer from a distant site or organ to the brain.

Etiology: Metastatic dissemination to the brain primarily occurs through hematogenous spread.

Epidemiology: Metastases to the brain accounts for approximately 15% to 25% of all intracranial tumors. Brain metastases may involve the supratentorial or infratentorial parenchyma, meninges, or calvarium. Most metastases to the brain parenchyma develop by hematogenous spread from primary lung, breast, gastrointestinal tract, kidney, and melanoma tumors. Metastases to the calvarium may result from breast and prostate cancers. Metastases to the meninges may result from bone or breast cancer.

Signs and Symptoms: Depending on the extent of involvement, the patient may present with seizures, signs of intracranial pressure, and loss in sensory/motor function.

Imaging Characteristics: MRI is more sensitive than CT for the detection of brain metastasis.

MRI and CT
- Show multiple discrete lesions with variable density along the gray-white matter interface.
- Show marked peripheral edema surrounding larger lesions.
- Postcontrast show ring-like enhancement on larger lesions.

MRI
- Lesions are hypointense to isointense to brain parenchyma on T1-weighted images.
- T2-weighted images show the lesions and surrounding edema as high-signal intensity.
- Postcontrast T1-weighted images demonstrate the lesion as hyperintense and the edema as hypointense.

Treatment: Usually patients with multiple metastatic lesions to the brain are treated with radiation therapy, while patients with a single metastatic lesion may undergo surgical removal of the lesion followed by radiation therapy.

Prognosis: Depends on the number and extent of metastatic lesions in the brain and if the patient has any evidence of other systemic cancer.

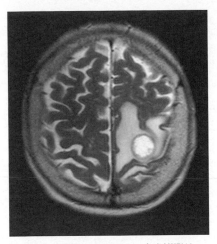

FIGURE 1. **Brain Metastasis.** Axial T2W image shows the left parietal mass with high central signal likely due to necrosis and high signal in the surrounding white matter due to vasogenic edema.

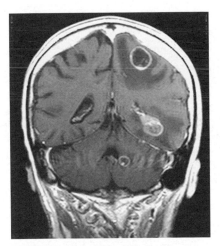

FIGURE 2. **Brain Metastasis.** Postcontrast T1W coronal MR shows multiple enhancing lesions with surrounding low-signal edema involving the gray-white junction, white matter, and cerebellum.

Craniopharyngioma

Description: Craniopharyngiomas are benign epithelial tumors that are almost always located in the suprasellar region and occasional in the intrasellar region.

Etiology: Craniopharyngiomas arise from squamous epithelial rests along the infundibulum of the hypophysis or Rathke pouch.

Epidemiology: These tumors have a bimodal age distribution. More than half occur in children and young adults, while the second, smaller peak occurs in the fifth and sixth decade of life. Approximately 40% of craniopharyngiomas occur in children between the ages of 8 and 12 years. Males and females are affected equally.

Signs and Symptoms: Patients may present with visual symptoms, obstructive hydrocephalus, and endocrine dysfunction.

Imaging Characteristics: Small tumors are typically well circumscribed, lobulated masses, while larger masses may be multicystic in appearance and invading the sella turcica. Craniopharyngiomas may present with calcification (90%), contrast enhance (90%), and cystic (85%), and measure between 2 and 6 cm in size (75%).

CT
- Lobulated solid and cystic suprasellar mass.
- Calcification seen in approximately 90% of pediatric tumors; adults 30% to 40%.
- Contrast enhancement of solid portions and periphery.

MRI
- Appearance may be extremely variable, with most showing low signal on T1-weighted images and bright on T2-weighted images.
- Solid portions of the tumor usually enhance with contrast.
- Cystic areas may be hyperintense on T1-weighted images.
- FLAIR images appear with high signal.

Treatment: Surgery is most commonly performed; however, the tumors may become so large that they are impossible to excise. Radiation therapy may also be used. Recurrence is common.

Prognosis: Surgical resection followed by radiation supports a 10-year survival rate of 78%.

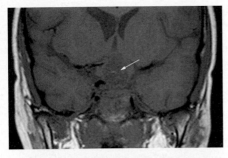

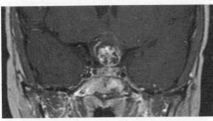

FIGURE 1. Craniopharyngioma. Coronal T1W MR image shows a low-signal suprasellar mass (arrow) with small focus of increased signal which enhances with contrast.

FIGURE 2. Craniopharyngioma. Postcontrast T1W coronal MR.

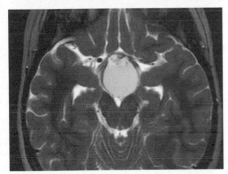

FIGURE 3. Craniopharyngioma. T2W axial image shows high signal within the cystic component of the mass. The punctate areas of low signal are due to calcification.

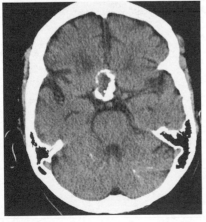

FIGURE 4. Craniopharyngioma. Axial NECT shows dense calcifications within a suprasellar mass consistent with a craniopharyngioma.

Ependymoma

Description: An ependymoma is an intracranial glioma which arises from the ependymal cells which line the ventricle system and central canal of the spinal cord.

Etiology: Unknown.

Epidemiology: Most commonly seen in the fourth ventricle. This is the third most common pediatric tumor. Posterior fossa (infratentorial) ependymomas make up approximately 10% to 15% of all pediatric tumors affecting the CNS and about 3% to 5% of all intracranial tumors in children 1 to 6 years of age.

Signs and Symptoms: Headaches, nausea, vomiting, ataxia, and vertigo.

Imaging Characteristics:

CT
- Hydrocephalus is seen in most cases.
- Hyperdense enhancement with IV contrast.
- Calcification, cysts, and edema may be seen in approximately 50% of cases.

MRI
- Appear hypointense to isointense on T1-weighted images.
- Appear hyperintense on T2-weighted images.
- Appear hyperintense with gadolinium.

Treatment: Surgical intervention to remove as much of the tumor as possible. Conventional radiation therapy and stereotactic radiosurgery may also be helpful.

Prognosis: Five-year survival is approximately 50%.

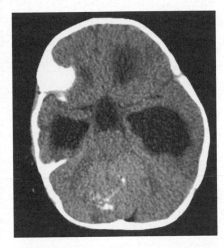

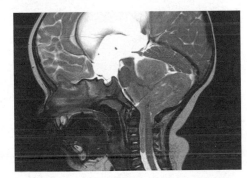

FIGURE 1. **Ependymoma.** Axial NECT shows a large mass with calcifications arising from the fourth ventricle and extending posteriorly. There is also hydrocephalus due to obstruction of cerebral spinal fluid (CSF) flow by the mass.

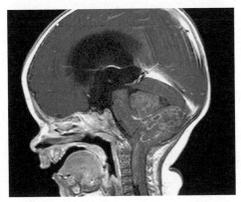

FIGURE 2. **Ependymoma.** Sagittal T2W image shows the large irregular mass arising from the fourth ventricle, compressing the cerebellum and herniating down the spinal canal. There is also severe hydrocephalus due to obstruction of CSF flow.

FIGURE 3. **Ependymoma.** Postcontrast T1W sagittal image shows irregular enhancement of the mass.

Glioblastoma Multiforme

Description: According to the WHO classification, a glioblastoma multiforme is also known as an astrocytoma Grade IV tumor. This rapid growing, highly malignant tumor is predominantly located in the intercerebral hemispheres, though similar lesions may occur in the brainstem, cerebellum, or spinal cord. It spreads by direct extension and can cross from one cerebral hemisphere to the other through connecting white matter tracts such as the corpus callosum.

Etiology: Unknown.

Epidemiology: The glioblastoma multiforme is the most common primary intracranial tumor. It typically appears between 45 and 60 years of age. Males are slightly more affected than females.

Signs and Symptoms: Patients may present with nausea and vomiting, headaches, papilledema, change in mental status, seizures, and speech and sensory disturbances.

Imaging Characteristics: These tumors are located in the white matter of the cerebral hemisphere and will appear heterogeneous, with edema and mass effect.

CT
- Nodular-rim enhancement with IV contrast demonstrates a necrotic tissue center.
- Edema is generally present.

MRI
- T1-weighted images present as mixed signal intensity.
- T2-weighted images demonstrate an increased signal (hyperintense) indicating a tumor and edema.
- T1-weighted contrast-enhanced images will demonstrate nodular-rim enhancement, the edema, and necrotic tissue as hypointense.

Treatment: Surgical resection (if operable), radiation therapy, and chemotherapy are currently the methods for treating glioblastoma multiforme.

Prognosis: Poor prognosis. The 1-year and 2-year survival rate is approximately 50% and 15%, respectively.

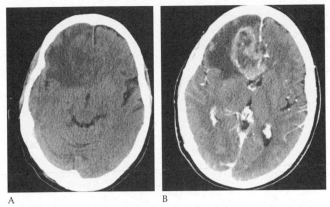

A   B

FIGURE 1. Glioblastoma Multiforme. Pre- (A) and postcontrast (B) axial CT images show a large peripherally enhancing centrally necrotic mass in the right frontal lobe which is extending across the white matter tracts of the anterior corpus callosum. Note the surrounding edema and mass effect resulting in midline shift.

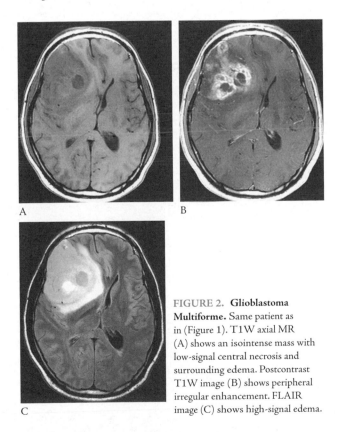

A   B

C   **FIGURE 2. Glioblastoma Multiforme.** Same patient as in (Figure 1). T1W axial MR (A) shows an isointense mass with low-signal central necrosis and surrounding edema. Postcontrast T1W image (B) shows peripheral irregular enhancement. FLAIR image (C) shows high-signal edema.

Lipoma

Description: A benign fatty tumor.

Etiology: Unknown.

Epidemiology: Incidence of less than 1% of primary intracranial tumors. May appear at any age. Are usually located in the midline (80% to 95%).

Signs and Symptoms: Asymptomatic, usually discovered as an incidental finding. Do not increase in size.

Imaging Characteristics:

CT
- Hypodense appearance. Do not enhance with contrast.

MRI
- Hyperintense on T1-weighted images.
- Hypointense on T2-weighted images.
- Hyperintense on T2-weighted images indicate either fat or subacute blood.
- Fat suppression images will differentiate between fat and blood.

Treatment: No treatment may be required.

Prognosis: Unless the lipoma is positioned in a life-threatening location, the patient's prognosis is unaffected.

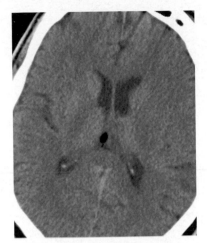

FIGURE 1. **Lipoma.** Axial NECT shows a small, very low-attenuation mass in the midline consistent with a lipoma.

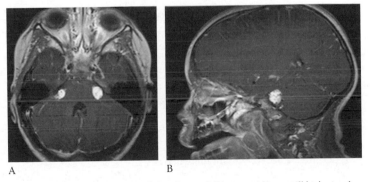

A   B

FIGURE 2. **Lipoma.** T1W axial (A) and sagittal (B) images show small high-signal-intensity masses in both cerebellopontine angles.

Medulloblastoma

Description: Medulloblastomas are rapid growing, highly malignant tumors arising in the posterior medullary velum.

Etiology: Arise from the embryonal cell rests in the germinative zone of the posterior medullary velum, a midline structure that contributes to the roof of the fourth ventricle.

Epidemiology: These tumors are the most common posterior fossa neoplasm in pediatric patients and account for approximately 20% of all primary brain tumors in the pediatric population. There is a bimodal incidence, showing a major peak in children between 5 and 8 years of age and a second smaller peak between 20 and 30 years of age. Seen more commonly in males than females at a ratio of 2:1.

Signs and Symptoms: Patients may experience hydrocephalus-like signs and symptoms such as increased intracranial pressure (ICP), ataxia, and nystagmus, and a herniation of the cerebellar tonsils can cause neck stiffness.

Imaging Characteristics:

CT
- Noncontrast study is hyperdense, in the midline, displacing the fourth ventricle.
- Enhances with IV contrast.

MRI
- T1-weighted images range from hypointense to isointense to gray matter.
- Hyperintense on T2-weighted images.

Treatment: Methods of treatment may include surgery resection, radiation therapy, and multiagent chemotherapy.

Prognosis: Good to poor prognosis depending on the patient's age, tumor location, and amount of tumor resected. Favorable prognostic factors include an age greater than 2 years, undisseminated local disease, and greater than 75% of the tumor resected.

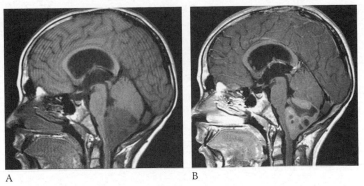

A   B

FIGURE 1. **Medulloblastoma.** Sagittal T1W image (A) shows a large low-signal fourth ventricular mass with multiple cystic areas. The solid component enhances with gadolinium (B). Also note the hydrocephalus due to obstruction of CSF flow.

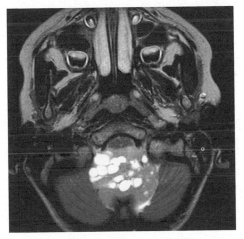

FIGURE 2. **Medulloblastoma.** Axial T2W image shows hyperintense cystic areas within the mass.

Meningioma

Description: Meningiomas are the most common benign intracranial neoplasms, and the second most common primary tumor affecting the central nervous system. Meningiomas are characteristically a hard, slow-growing, usually highly vascular tumor occurring mainly along the meningeal vessels and superior longitudinal sinus. They invade the dura and skull and lead to erosion and thinning of the skull. In some cases, these tumors may also grow on the spine.

Etiology: Arise from the meninges.

Epidemiology: Meningiomas are primarily adult tumors. They account for approximately 20% of all primary brain tumors. The peak incidence is between 40 and 60 years of age. Females are slightly more affected than males by a ratio of 3:2. The majority of meningiomas (90%) are intracranial, and 90% of these are supratentorial.

Signs and Symptoms: The signs and symptoms a patient may present depends on the location and size of the tumor. However, headaches, seizures, nausea and vomiting, and changes in mental status may be seen.

Imaging Characteristics:

CT

- Noncontrast study demonstrates a slightly hyperdense extraaxial mass.
- IV contrast study demonstrates marked enhancement.
- Calcification is seen in 20% to 25% of cases.

MRI

- T1-weighted images demonstrate an isointense to slightly hypointense mass.
- T1-weighted images greatly enhance following gadolinium administration.
- T2-weighted images demonstrate a meningioma as isointense to slight hypointense.

Treatment: Surgical resection is used to remove this benign mass. Radiotherapy may be useful when complete surgical removal is not possible or the meningioma recurs.

Prognosis: Completely resected meningiomas provide an excellent prognosis with 10-year survival rate of 80% to 90%.

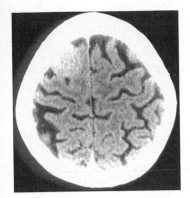

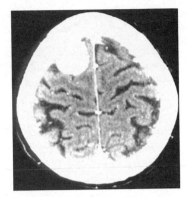

FIGURE 1. Meningioma. Noncontrast CT shows round, high-density mass over the convexity of the right parietal lobe.

FIGURE 2. Meningioma. Postcontrast CT image shows a round, markedly contrast-enhancing mass over the convexity of the right parietal lobe.

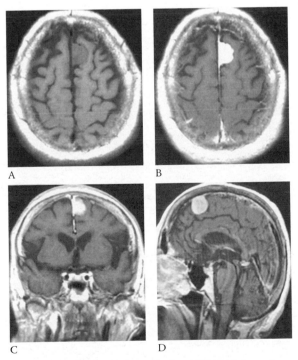

A

B

C

D

FIGURE 3. Meningioma. T1-weighted axial MR image shows an isointense left parasagittal meningioma (A) and postcontrast T1-weighted images in the axial (B), coronal (C), and sagittal (D) planes.

Oligodendroglioma

Description: Oligodendrogliomas are primary glial brain tumors. They tend to be slow-growing, solid, and calcified tumors. They are primarily found in the supratentorial white matter.

Etiology: Unknown.

Epidemiology: These tumors represent about 5% of all intracranial gliomas and 5% of all intracranial neoplasms. Males are more affected than females by a ratio of 2:1. These tumors may occur at any age; however, the average age when diagnosed is between 40 and 50 years.

Signs and Symptoms: Seizures, headaches, change in behavior, weakness, or paralysis.

Imaging Characteristics: MRI is the preferred imaging modality.

CT
- Mass appears hypodense with moderate swelling.
- Calcification is commonly seen.
- Edema is typically not seen.
- Enhancement with IV contrast is variable.

MRI
- Appear hypointense on T1-weighted images.
- Appear hyperintense on T2-weighted and FLAIR images except in areas of calcification.
- Low-grade oligodendroglioma typically does not enhance with IV contrast, while an anaplastic oligodendroglioma does enhance.

Treatment: Surgery, radiation therapy, and chemotherapy.

Prognosis: Five-year survival is 50%.

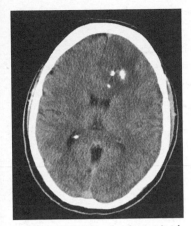

FIGURE 1. Oligodendroglioma. Axial NECT shows an ill-defined partially calcified mass with surrounding edema in the left frontal lobe white matter.

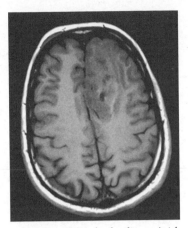

FIGURE 2. Oligodendroglioma. Axial T1W image shows an ill-defined mass in the left frontal lobe that is isointense to the surrounding gray matter.

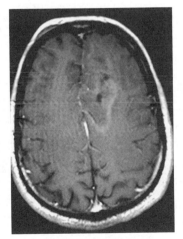

FIGURE 3. Oligodendroglioma. Postgadolinium T1W image shows minimal peripheral enhancement of the mass.

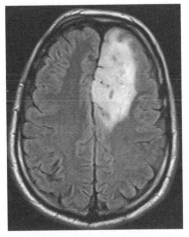

FIGURE 4. Oligodendroglioma. Axial FLAIR shows a heterogeneous, hyperintense mass in the left frontal lobe which is fairly well circumscribed with some mild surrounding edema.

Pituitary Adenoma

Description: Pituitary adenomas are also classified as either functioning or nonfunctioning, depending on their ability to secrete hormones.

Etiology: The exact cause is unknown; however, there is a predisposition that pituitary tumors are inherited through an autosomal dominant trait.

Epidemiology: Pituitary adenomas constitute 10% of all intracranial neoplasms and are the most common primary neoplasm found in the sellar region. Occur in both male and females equally during the third and fourth decades of life.

Signs and Symptoms: Patients may present with frontal headaches, visual symptoms, increased intracranial pressure, personality changes, seizures, rhinorrhea, and pituitary apoplexy secondary to hemorrhagic infarction of the adenoma.

Imaging Characteristics: Adenomas that measure less than 10 mm are defined as microadenomas, while those measuring greater than 10 mm are defined as macroadenomas.

CT
- Focal region of hypodensity within the gland.
- Following contrast enhancement the tumor will be isodense to the normal pituitary gland.

MRI
- T1-weighted images appear as a region of hypointensity within the gland.
- T1-weighted contrast-enhanced images appear hyperintense.
- T2-weighted images appear with a variable signal that is unpredictable.

Treatment: Methods may include transsphenoidal pituitary resection, cryohypophysectomy, pituitary irradiation, or bromocriptine.

Prognosis: The patient's prognosis is ranked from fair to good, depending on the extent the tumor spreads outside the sella turcica.

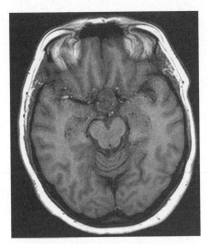

FIGURE 1. Pituitary Adenoma. Axial T1W MR shows a sellar mass that is isointense to the surrounding gray matter.

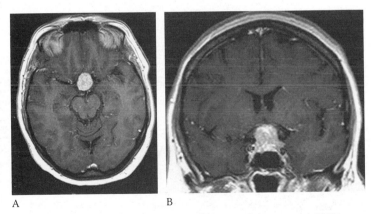

A   B

FIGURE 2. Pituitary Adenoma. Axial (A) and coronal (B) postcontrast T1W images show heterogeneous enhancement of the mass consistent with a pituitary macroadenoma.

BRAIN
CONGENITAL

Agenesis of the Corpus Callosum

Description: A partial or complete absence of the corpus callosum.

Etiology: Agenesis of the corpus callosum is caused by an insult that has occurred embryologically prior to the 10th week of gestation.

Epidemiology: Anomalies (agenesis) of the corpus callosum occur between 10 and 18 weeks of gestation. Males and females are equally affected.

Signs and Symptoms: Patients may present asymptomatic; however, in many cases there are developmental abnormalities present.

Imaging Characteristics: CT and MRI demonstrate an elevated third ventricle, noticeable separation of the lateral ventricles, partial or complete absences of the corpus callosum, and dysplasia of the cerebellum.

Treatment: There is no treatment for this condition; however, conditions such as hydrocephalus may require treatment.

Prognosis: Depends on other extenuating circumstances that may be related to other developmental abnormalities.

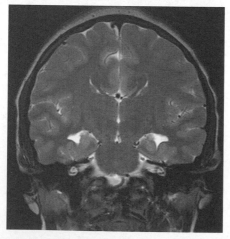

FIGURE 1. **Agenesis of the Corpus Callosum.** Coronal T2W image shows agenesis of the corpus callosum with widely spaced lateral ventricle and continuity of the third ventricle with the interhemispheric fissure.

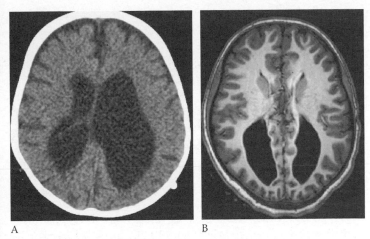

A   B

FIGURE 2. Agenesis of the Corpus Callosum. Axial CT (A) and axial T1W MR (B) show enlarged and parallel lateral ventricles with a "race car" configuration and no corpus callosum.

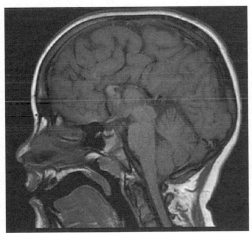

FIGURE 3. Agenesis of the Corpus Callosum. Sagittal T1W image shows congenital absence of the corpus callosum with radially oriented gyri and the absence of the cingulate gyrus.

Arachnoid Cyst

Description: Arachnoid cysts are benign cerebrospinal fluid-filled sacs which may be located in relationship to the arachnoid membrane. They do not communicate with the ventricular system.

Etiology: They are usually congenital; however, they may result from a posttraumatic or postsurgical event.

Epidemiology: They make up about 1% of all intracranial masses. Approximately 50% to 60% occur in the middle fossa. Males are four times more likely than females to have an arachnoid cyst.

Signs and Symptoms: Depending on the size and location of the cyst, they may go undetected. Large cysts may cause headaches, impairment of vision, seizures, increased collection of CSF, increased intracranial pressure (ICP), delay in mental and physical development, and altered behavior.

Imaging Characteristics:

MRI and CT
- Extraaxial benign-appearing CSF-filled cystic mass.
- Most common supratentorial locations include: (1) middle cranial fossa; (2) parasellar cisterns; and (3) subarachnoid space over the convexities.

Treatment: Surgery is used to relieve symptoms. A shunt may be used to reduce the ICP by draining the CSF into the peritoneum.

Prognosis: Good, arachnoid cysts are benign and treatable.

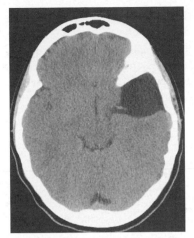

FIGURE 1. Arachnoid Cyst. Axial NECT shows a CSF density well circumscribed extra-axial fluid collection in the left middle cranial fossa with posterior displacement of the left temporal lobe.

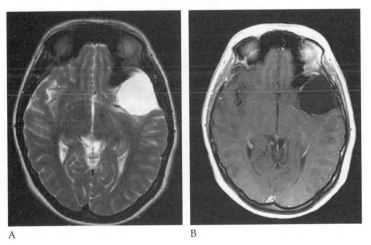

A   B

FIGURE 2. Arachnoid Cyst. Axial T2W (A) and T1W C+ (B) images follow the signal characteristics of the CSF.

Crainosynostosis

Description: Crainosynostosis is a congenital condition in which one or more of the cranial sutures fuse prematurely. The three most common types are: (1) scaphocephaly (sagittal)—the most common type; (2) plagiocephaly; and (3) trionocephaly.

Etiology: Unknown.

Epidemiology: Occurs in 1 out of 2000 live births. Males are affected twice more often than females.

Signs and Symptoms: An absence of the "soft spot" (fontanelle), a hard ridge along the affected suture, unusual head shape, or abnormal head size may be indicators for this condition. An increase in the intracranial pressure (ICP) may occur.

Imaging Characteristics:

CT
- Three-dimensional imaging is beneficial to see bony detail.
- Bone windows show fusion of sutures.

MRI
- Useful for long-term follow-up.

Treatment: Craniofacial surgery may be required.

Prognosis: Depends on the degree of this congenital condition.

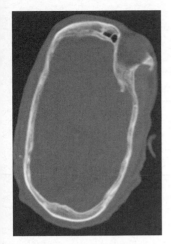

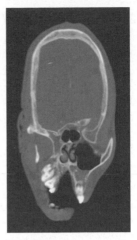

FIGURE 1. Crainosynostosis.
Axial NECT shows elongation
of the calvarium in the antero-
posterior dimension and narrowing
in the transverse dimension.

FIGURE 2. Crainosynostosis.
Coronal NECT shows
premature complete fusion of
the sagittal suture.

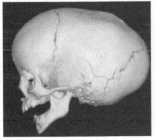

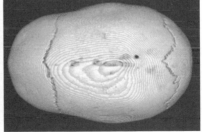

A   B

FIGURE 3. Crainosynostosis. Lateral 3D reconstructed image (A) and above view
(B) image of the skull show complete fusion of the sagittal suture and elongation of the
skull in the AP dimension.

Dandy-Walker Syndrome

Description: Dandy-Walker syndrome is a noncommunicating type of hydrocephalus, which results from a partial dysgenesis of the vermis and a remnant fourth ventricle that communicates with a retrocerebellar cyst that is also known as a Blake pouch (see the section Hydrocephalus).

Etiology: An atresia of the foramen of Magendie and foramina of Luschka of the fourth ventricle.

Epidemiology: Represents approximately 2% of all cases of hydrocephalus. Occurs in 1 per 25,000 to 30,000 births and is usually diagnosed by 1 year of age. Males and females are equally affected. Associated with hydrocephalus in 80% of cases and agenesis of the corpus callosum in 20% of the cases.

Signs and Symptoms: Related to hydrocephalus and other associated anomalies.

Imaging Characteristics: Appears as a massively dilated fourth ventricle expanding into the posterior fossa demonstrating hydrocephalus. Both CT and MRI images demonstrate a massively dilated fourth ventricle, expanded posterior fossa with an inferior hypoplastic vermis.

CT
- Hypodense CSF-filled space located in the posterior fossa involving the fourth ventricle.

MRI
- Hypointense on T1-weighted images.
- Hyperintense on T2-weighted images.

Treatment: Surgical intervention and shunting the excess CSF into the right atrium or the peritoneal cavity.

Prognosis: Depends on other neurologic complications; however, surgical intervention and shunting the excess CSF into the right atrium or into the peritoneal cavity will control the Dandy-Walker syndrome.

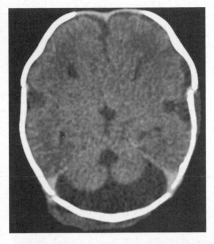

FIGURE 1. **Dandy-Walker Syndrome.** Axial NECT shows a large posterior fossa with a CSF density cyst, hypoplastic cerebellar hemispheres, and absence of the vermis.

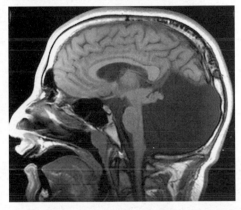

FIGURE 2. **Dandy-Walker Syndrome.** Sagittal T1W image shows a massively dilated fourth ventricle, expanded posterior fossa, high-riding torcula, and hypoplastic cerebellum.

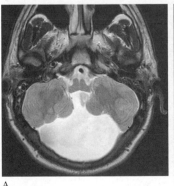

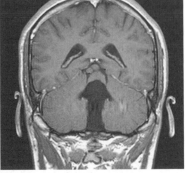

A   B

FIGURE 3. **Dandy-Walker Syndrome.** Axial T2W (A) and coronal T1W (B) show absence of the cerebellar vermis.

Encephalocele

Description: Encephaloceles result from a herniation of the brain or meninges, or both, through a skull defect. The hernia may be a small CSF-filled meningeal sac or a large cyst-like structure that may exceed the size of the head. It may be covered with skin and/or membrane of varying thickness, and may contain the pons, midbrain, and vermis structures. The herniated portion of the brain is nonfunctioning.

Etiology: Results from a congenital defect or a trauma opening in the skull.

Epidemiology: Newborns are mostly affected. Encephaloceles account for 10% to 20% of craniospinal malformations. The incidence rate is approximately 1 to 3 per 10,000. The skull defect is commonly found in the occipital region (71%), parietal region (10%), and throughout the skull base (18%).

Signs and Symptoms: Patients may present with hydrocephalus, developmental delay, motor weakness and/or spasticity, ataxia, mental retardation, microcephaly, seizures, and visual problems.

Imaging Characteristics:

CT
- Osseous defect is best evaluated with CT.

MRI
- Provides excellent delineation of the CSF and soft tissue brain components of an encephalocele.

Treatment: In cases involving hydrocephalus, shunting CSF from the brain may be necessary.

Prognosis: The prognosis of fetuses with an encephalocele is variable depending on the presence of brain in the sac, hydrocephalus, and microcephaly. With brain involvement the prognosis may be quite poor.

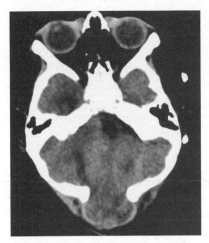

FIGURE 1. Encephalocele. Axial NECT shows a small amount of brain protruding posteriorly through a midline defect in the occipital bone.

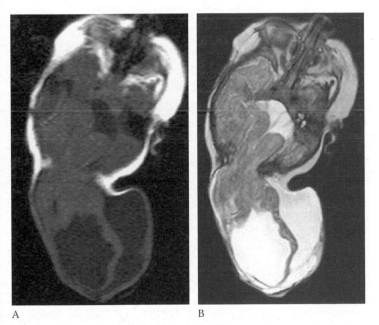

A   B

FIGURE 2. Encephalocele. Axial T1W (A) and T2W (B) images showing herniation of the brain through a defect in the posterior skull.

Hydrocephalus

Description: Hydrocephalus is an enlargement of the ventricular system of the brain also known in layman terms as "water on the brain." There are two types of hydrocephalus: noncommunicating and communicating. Hydrocephalus may result from an excessive amount of cerebral spinal fluid production, inadequate reabsorption of CSF, or an obstruction of the flow of the CSF from one or more of the ventricles.

In the noncommunicating type of hydrocephalus, the flow of the cerebral spinal fluid (CSF) from the ventricular system into the subarachnoid space is obstructed by a mass-occupying lesion, congenital narrowing of the aqueduct of Sylvius, or associated with a meningomyelocele.

The communicating type of hydrocephalus may result from an overproduction of CSF in the choroid plexus, or inadequate reabsorption of CSF by the arachnoid villi.

Note:
1. In the Dandy-Walker syndrome, an atresia of the foramen of Magendie results in an enlarged fourth ventricle.
2. Normal-pressure hydrocephalus typically affects adults with progressive dementia.

Etiology: Hydrocephalus may result from: (1) an excessive amount of CSF production; (2) inadequate reabsorption of CSF by the arachnoid villi; or (3) an obstruction of the outflow of the CSF from one or more of the ventricles.

Epidemiology: This congenital defect may also be associated with a history of a meningomyelocele.

Signs and Symptoms: Patient may present with increase in the circumference of the head, behavioral changes such as irritability and lethargy, seizures and vomiting, or a change in appetite.

Imaging Characteristics: MRI is the better modality for the evaluation of hydrocephalus.

CT
◆ Noncontrast study demonstrates enlarged ventricles (hypodense).

MRI
◆ T1-weighted images demonstrate the enlarged CSF-filled ventricles as hypointense.
◆ T1-weighted contrast-enhanced sequence should be performed to rule out intracranial mass if indicated.
◆ T2-weighted images demonstrate the enlarged CSF-filled ventricles as hyperintense.

Treatment: Shunting the excess CSF into the right atrium or into the peritoneal cavity.

Prognosis: Good, following shunting procedure.

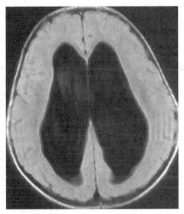

FIGURE 1. **Hydrocephalus.** T1-weighted axial MRI shows markedly dilated lateral ventricles with low-signal CSF.

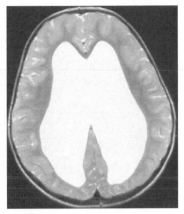

FIGURE 2. **Hydrocephalus.** T2-weighted axial MRI shows high-signal CSF of the markedly dilated lateral ventricles.

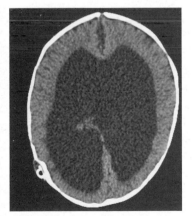

FIGURE 3. **Hydrocephalus.** Axial NECT shows markedly dilated lateral ventricles.

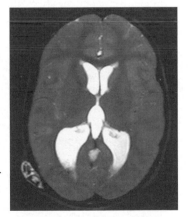

FIGURE 4. **Hydrocephalus.** T2W axial image shows high-signal CSF within markedly dilated lateral ventricles as a result of a shunt malfunction (fluid leaking around shunt in right parieto-occipital soft tissues).

Neurofibromatosis (NF1)

Description: Neurofibromatosis type 1 (NF1) is a multisystem generic disorder which causes tumors (neurofibromas) to grow in the nervous system.

Etiology: Hereditary.

Epidemiology: The incidence of NF1 is 1 in 2500 to 4000 individuals.

Signs and Symptoms: The following are diagnostic findings for NF1.

- Six or more café-au-lait spots (light brown spots) on the skin measuring 5 mm in diameter in children or more than 15 mm in adolescents and adults.
- Two or more neurofibromas.
- Freckling in the area of the armpit or groin.
- Familiar history of NF1.

Imaging Characteristics: MRI is the imaging modality of choice.

CT
- Bony erosion may be seen.
- Hydrocephalus may be seen.
- Calcification, especially at the vertex, may be seen.
- Demonstrate solid fusiform and plexiform neurofibromas with attenuation values of 30 to 40 HU.
- Good to evaluate the chest, abdomen, and pelvis of NF1 patients.

MRI
- Intracranial nerve sheath tumors are isointense to brain tissue on T1-weighted and hyperintense on T2-weighted images.
- Tumors appear with a smooth margin.
- Enhance with gadolinium.
- Optic gliomas, most common intracranial tumor for NH1; other gliomas may be seen in other parts of the brain.
- Large tumor may be heterogeneous.

Treatment: Surgery as needed.

Prognosis: Patient usually lives a healthy life; however, overall life expectancy may be reduced by as much as 15 years mostly due to malignant tumors.

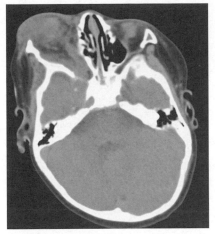

FIGURE 1. Neurofibromatosis (NF1).
Axial NECT shows a soft tissue density
infiltrative mass of the right orbit with moderate
exophthalmos.

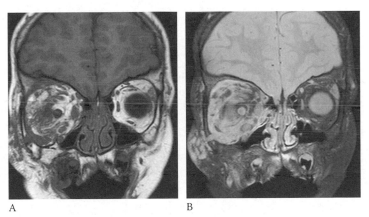

A   B

FIGURE 2. Neurofibromatosis (NF1). Coronal T1W image (A) shows low-signal-
intensity mass within the right orbit which is bright on T2W images (B) consistent
with a plexiform neurofibroma.

Tuberous Sclerosis

Description: Tuberous sclerosis is a rare, multisystem genetic disease which causes benign tumors to grow in the brain and other organs of the body.

Etiology: About 50% are hereditary and 50% are sporadic.

Epidemiology: Prevalence rate is 1 in 6000 to 15,000 population. Most cases are diagnosed between the ages of 2 and 6 years.

Signs and Symptoms: Characteristic findings include seizures, mental retardation, and adenoma sebaceum.

Imaging Characteristics:

CT
- Used to identify tumors of the brain and abdomen.
- Shows calcified cortical tubers and subependymal nodules.
- Cortical tubers seen as low-attenuating peripheral lesion.
- Subependymal nodules usually found along the lateral ventricles.
- Tubers usually do not enhance.

MRI
- T1-weighted images may appear hyperintense in infants and hypointense in adults.
- T2-weighted images may appear hypointense in infants and hyperintense in adults.
- FLAIR images are good for seeing small tubers.

Treatment: Medical care is usually focused on controlling seizures. Surgical intervention as needed.

Prognosis: Depends on the severity of the symptoms.

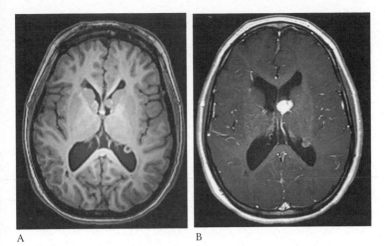

A   B

FIGURE 1. Tuberous Sclerosis. PD axial (A) and postcontrast T1W (B) contrast shows an enhancing left subependymal giant cell astrocytoma in the foramen of Monroe and an enhancing subependymal nodule in the trigone of the left lateral ventricle.

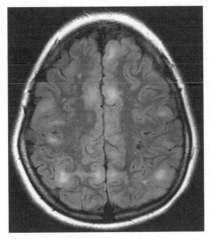

FIGURE 2. Tuberous Sclerosis. Axial FLAIR shows multiple hyperintense cortical and subcortical nodules and small low-signal-intensity cystic lesions.

BRAIN

PHAKOMATOSIS

Sturge-Weber Syndrome

Description: Sturge-Weber syndrome (encephalotrigeminal angiomatosis) is a congenital disorder characterized by localized atrophy and calcification of the cerebral cortex with an ipsilateral port-wine colored facial nevus in the area of the trigeminal nerve distribution.

Etiology: Hereditary disorder attributed to autosomal dominant and autosomal recessive patterns.

Epidemiology: Incidence is 1 per 1000 patients in mental institutions.

Signs and Symptoms: Patients may present with port-wine stain, seizure disorder, hemiatrophy, hemianopsia, mental retardation, and glaucoma.

Imaging Characteristics:

CT
- Cerebral atrophy may be seen.
- Calcified areas of the brain will appear hyperdense.

MRI
- Cerebral atrophy is best seen on T1-weighted images.
- Lower (hypointense) signal may be present in calcified areas of the brain.
- FLAIR images are used to demonstrate leptomeningeal (pia mater and arachnoid) abnormality as a hyperintense signal.

Treatment: Symptomatic treatment for the above-mentioned conditions.

Prognosis: Most cases are considered to be mild and life expectancy is usually normal.

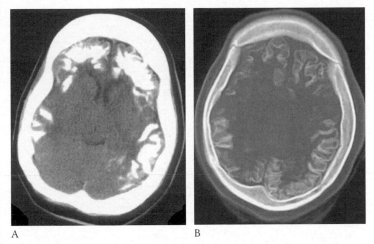

A   B

FIGURE 1. Sturge-Weber Syndrome. Noncontrast CT images of the brain (A) and bone window (B) demonstrate bilateral frontal and parietal cortical calcifications.

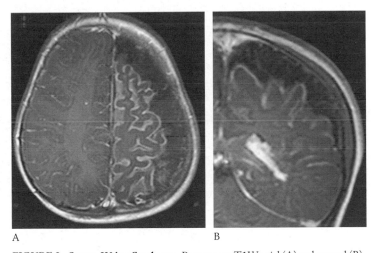

A   B

FIGURE 2. Sturge-Weber Syndrome. Postcontrast T1W axial (A) and coronal (B) images show cerebral atrophy.

Von Hippel-Lindau Disease

Description: An autosomal dominant (hereditary) condition characterized by angiomas of the retina and cerebellum, visceral cysts and malignancies, seizures and mental retardation.

Etiology: Hereditary disorder.

Epidemiology: Prevalence is estimated at 1 in 35,000 to 40,000 of the population. There is no predilection toward males or females.

Signs and Symptoms: Patients typically become symptomatic in their third or fourth decade of life. Characterized by retinal angiomas, hemangioblastomas of the cerebellum and spinal cord, cystic disease of the kidney, pancreas, and liver, and a risk of malignancy involving the kidneys, adrenal glands, or pancreas. Patients may experience seizures and mental retardation.

Imaging Characteristics:

MRI
- Tumors within the CNS appear as isointense to hypointense on T1-weighted images.
- T2-weighted images present the tumors as hyperintense.
- T1-weighted images with contrast demonstrate the tumor as hyperintense (the most sensitive means of detecting the CNS tumor).

Treatment: Symptomatic treatment for the above-mentioned conditions and surgical intervention of tumors where and when appropriate.

Prognosis: Varies depending on degree of symptoms and if cancer is detected. There is no known cure for this hereditary disease. Death is usually associated with complications of brain tumors or renal cancer.

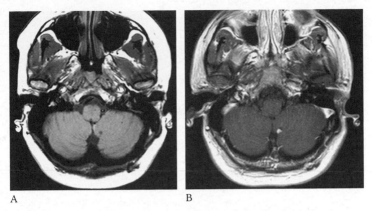

A   B

FIGURE 1. Von Hippel-Lindau Disease. Axial T1W (A) shows a small hypointense nodule in the medial aspect of the left cerebellar hemisphere which enhances with contrast administration T1W with gadolinium (B).

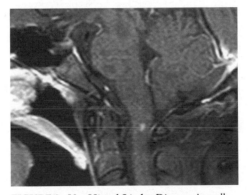

FIGURE 2. Von Hippel-Lindau Disease. A small enhancing nodule is seen on a sagittal T1W image with gadolinium. These are likely hemangioblastomas in this patient with Von Hippel-Lindau (VHL) disease.

BRAIN
VASCULAR DISEASE

Arteriovenous Malformation

Description: An arteriovenous malformation (AVM) is the most common type of vascular malformation and is characterized by direct artery-to-vein communication without an intervening capillary bed.

Etiology: An AVM is a congenital lesion, which is the result of abnormal fetal development at approximately 3-week gestation.

Epidemiology: Males generally present during middle age and are slightly more affected than females. Between 80% and 90% are located in the cerebrum, 10% and 20% located in the posterior fossa.

Signs and Symptoms: Clinical presentation depends on the location and size of the AVM with most present between the second and third decade of life. By the age of 50 years, 80% to 90% are symptomatic. Hemorrhage will be present in about 50% of the cases. Other symptoms include seizures and headaches.

Imaging Characteristics: Appears as a collection of "worms."

CT
- Isodense to slightly hyperdense without contrast enhancement.
- Calcification in 25% to 30%.
- Atrophy.
- Hyperdense serpentine-appearing vessels with contrast enhancement.

MRI
- T1- and T2-weighted images demonstrate serpentine-appearing vessels with signal variations (flow void) in the vessels.

Treatment: Depends on the age and general health of the patient. Endovascular embolization therapy, surgery intervention, stereotactic radiotherapy, or a combination of the above is useful in treating an AVM.

Prognosis: The mortality rate is approximately 10% when a hemorrhage is present.

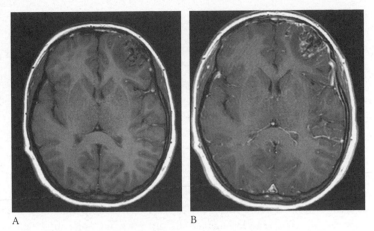

A   B

FIGURE 1. Arteriovenous Malformation. Axial T1W pre- (A) and postcontrast (B) enhanced images show a left frontal lobe mass with surrounding edema, minimal peripheral enhancement, and "worm"-like flow voids.

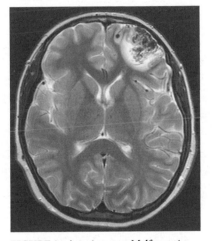

FIGURE 2. Arteriovenous Malformation. T2W axial image shows hyperintense edema around the mass of "worm-like" flow voids.

Intracranial Aneurysm

Description: An intracranial aneurysm is a localized dilation of a cerebral artery. The most common form is the berry aneurysm, a saclike outpouching usually arising at an arterial junction in the circle of Willis. Cerebral aneurysms often rupture and result in a subarachnoid hemorrhage.

Etiology: Weakening of the arterial wall may result from hemodynamic stresses. As an example, hypertension and atherosclerosis may restrict blood flow, thus increasing blood pressure against an arterial wall, stretching it like an overblown balloon, and making it likely to rupture. There is an increased incidence with polycystic kidney disease, aortic coarctation, and family history.

Epidemiology: Incidence rate is slightly higher in women than men. The peak age of occurrence is between 40 and 60 years. Anterior circulation is affected 90% of the time, while the vertebrobasilar circulation is affected only 10%.

Signs and Symptoms: Intracranial aneurysms may go undetected until they rupture; however, a very large nonruptured aneurysm can mimic the signs and symptoms of a tumor. If the aneurysm ruptures, they usually present as a subarachnoid hemorrhage. Signs and symptoms may vary depending on the location and severity of the ruptured aneurysm. Other common signs and symptoms may include headaches, nausea and vomiting, hemiparesis or motor deficit, nuchal rigidity, loss of consciousness, and coma.

Imaging Characteristics: Conventional angiography is the gold standard for the diagnosis of aneurysms.

CT

- In patients with ruptured intracranial aneurysm, a noncontrast study demonstrates a subarachnoid hemorrhage in the basilar cisterns as hyperdense in approximately 95% of the cases.
- Contrast-enhanced CT may show very large aneurysms.

MRI

- T1- and T2-weighted images appear with variable intensities (flow void).
- Magnetic resonance angiography (MRA) can diagnose most large aneurysms (>5 mm).

Treatment: Surgical intervention is best accomplished by a small metal clip or ligation around the neck of the aneurysm. Neuroradiologic intervention techniques also available for treatment of intracranial aneurysms include Guglielmi detachable (GD) coils.

Prognosis: In event that the aneurysm ruptures, the prognosis may be determined by the severity of the initial hemorrhage, rebleeding of the aneurysm, and vasospasm.

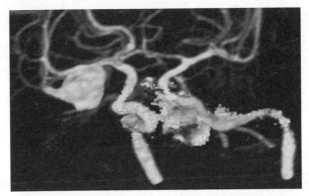

FIGURE 1. **Intracranial Aneurysm.** Computed tomography angiography (CTA) 3D reconstruction shows a large right M1 middle cerebral artery (MCA) aneurysm.

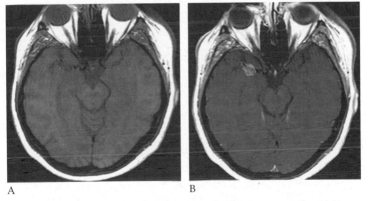

A   B

FIGURE 2. **Intracranial Aneurysm.** Axial T1W pre- (A) and postcontrast (B) enhanced images show an enhancing mass in the region of the right MCA.

Intracerebral Hemorrhage (Hemorrhagic Stroke)

Description: Intracerebral hemorrhages (ICH) occur when blood escapes from a ruptured vessel in the brain.

Etiology: Results from a rupturing of a blood vessel, usually an artery, within the brain. Hemorrhagic infarcts are frequently associated with hypertension, arteriosclerosis, or an aneurysm. Other factors may include trauma, neoplasms (primary or metastases), or drug use such as cocaine, amphetamine, and phenylpropanolamine.

Epidemiology: Approximately 20% of all strokes are hemorrhagic.

Signs and Symptoms: Patient may present with paralysis, motor weakness, headaches, or loss of consciousness.

Imaging Characteristics: CT is the modality of choice for the diagnosis of an intracranial hemorrhage.

CT
- Hyperacute (<4 hours) hyperdense.
- Acute (24 to 72 hours) hyperdense.
- Early subacute (4 to 7 days) hyperdense.
- Late subacute (1 to 4 weeks) isodense.
- Chronic (≥2 weeks) hypodense.

MRI

	T1-Weighted Image	T2-Weighted Image
Acute (24 to 72 hours)	Isointense to hypointense	Hypointense
Early subacute (4 to 7 days)	Hyperintense	Hypointense
Late subacute (1 to 4 weeks)	Hyperintense	Hyperintense
Chronic (2 weeks or more)	Hypointense	Hypointense

Treatment: Directed at reducing intracranial pressure (ICP) and controlling recurrent bleeding. Emergent surgery may be necessary to remove hematoma.

Prognosis: Depends on the location and severity of the hemorrhage.

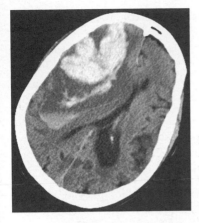

FIGURE 1. Intracerebral Hemorrhage. Axial NECT shows a large hyperdense region in the right parietal lobe consistent with acute hemorrhage. This is surrounded by low-attenuation cerebral edema. Note the mass effect and midline shift.

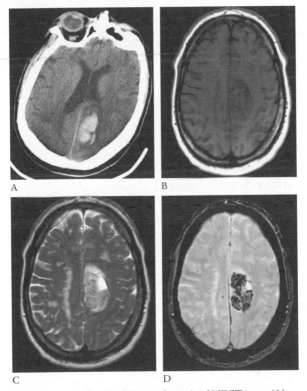

A

B

C

D

FIGURE 2. Intracerebral Hemorrhage. Axial NECT image (A) shows an acute hemorrhage in the left posterior parietal lobe. Note the blunting of the left ventricle. An axial T1W image (B) shows this area as isointense to hypointense. T2W axial image (C) shows the blood to be mildly hyperintense. Gradient echo axial MR (D) shows the blood products to be hypointense.

Ischemic Stroke (Cerebrovascular Accident)

Description: A cerebrovascular accident (CVA) or stroke occurs as a result of ischemia or hemorrhage. Cerebral ischemia is a reduction in the regional or global blood flow to the brain.

Etiology: Thromboembolic disease, usually as a result of atherosclerosis, is the primary cause of ischemic cerebrovascular disease. The source of emboli may vary and arise from arterial stenosis and occlusion, atherosclerotic debris, or from cardiac sources. Emboli from a cardiac source occur in about 15% to 20% of ischemic strokes.

Epidemiology: Approximately 80% to 85% of all strokes are ischemic. This is the third leading cause of death among Americans following cardiovascular disease and cancer. Males are affected approximately three times more than females. People over 65 years of age are at a greater risk. Black men are 1.5 times more at risk for having a stroke than white men.

Signs and Symptoms: Depends on the etiology, location of the ischemia, and the extent of damage to the brain cells.

Imaging Characteristics: MRI is more sensitive than CT; however, noncontrast CT is more efficient for the diagnosis of an acute stroke, to rule out hemorrhage.

CT

- Is useful in establishing the presence or absence of a hemorrhage and therefore prescribing a thrombolytic or anticoagulant treatment.
- Acute stage: Noncontrast study demonstrates a hyperdense middle cerebral artery, disappearing basal ganglia, and loss of insular cortex.
- Subacute stage: Demonstrates wedge-shaped area of low density involving both gray and white matter.

MRI

- May identify about 80% of strokes during the initial 24 hours.
- Acute stage: Vascular enhancement (slow flow) sign may be seen within 2 hours after ictus.
- Subacute stage: Parenchymal enhancement may appear hyperintense on T2-weighted images.
- Chronic stage: Appears hypointense on T1-weighted images and hyperintense on T2-weighted images. Chances of malacia with brain volume loss.
- Diffusion-weighted imaging (DWI) is more sensitive in showing an infarct within a few hours, as an area of increased signal.

Treatment: Depending on the time of onset, thrombolytic therapy may be helpful if administered within the first 3 hours following the initial onset of an ischemic stroke. Other methods of treatment may include anticoagulant therapy such as the use of heparin and warfarin or the administration of calcium channel blocking drugs.

Prognosis: Depends on the severity of the stroke. There is a 50% mortality rate within the first 24 hours following a stroke. Strokes affecting the posterior circulation have a higher mortality rate, but usually make a better recovery than hemispheric strokes.

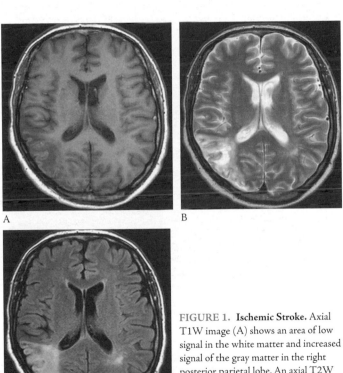

A

B

C

FIGURE 1. **Ischemic Stroke.** Axial T1W image (A) shows an area of low signal in the white matter and increased signal of the gray matter in the right posterior parietal lobe. An axial T2W image (B) shows increased signal in this area consistent with edema. FLAIR (C) shows increased signal in the white and gray matter in this region.

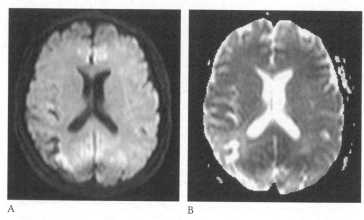

FIGURE 2. Ischemic Stroke. The portions of the area are bright on diffusion-weighted imaging (A), but this is also bright on the apparent diffusion coefficient (ADC) map (B) consistent with a subacute infarct.

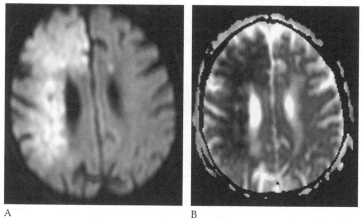

FIGURE 3. Ischemic Stroke. In an acute stroke the diffusion will be bright (A) and the ADC map will be dark (B).

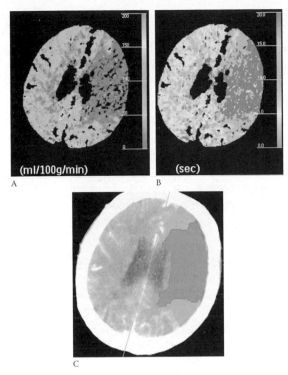

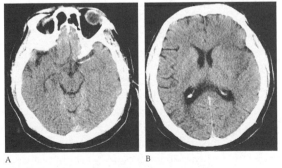

FIGURE 4. **Ischemic Stroke.** Same patient as in Figure 5 with
the left MCA stroke. Shows decreased cerebral perfusion to this
area (blue) (A). Mean transit time is prolonged (blue) (B).
In image (C) red represents an infarct; green represents the
penumbra of threatened (at risk) ischemic brain that may
potentially be saved with an intervention. (see Color Insert).

FIGURE 5. **Ischemic Stroke.** NECT axial image (A) shows a
hyperdense left MCA. There is decreased attenuation in the left
MCA territory (B) in the same patient and loss of the gray with
differentiation resulting in the "insular ribbon sign."

Neurovascular Compression Syndrome (NVCS)

Description: Neurovascular compression syndrome may also be referred to as vascular loop syndrome. This condition occurs where blood vessels come in direct contact with a cranial nerve producing a mechanical irritation of the cranial nerve.

Etiology: Two reasons appear to result in producing symptoms in patients. The first reason is mechanical irritation or compression of a cranial nerve (CN) by a blood vessel. Arteries are more likely to cause symptoms than veins, presumably due to the higher blood pressure and pulsatile motion. Second, the anatomical location of the neurovascular contact. The transition zone (TZ) of the cranial nerve seems to be the area of particular interest in producing symptoms associated with NVCS.

Epidemiology: The most common neurovascular compression syndromes include (1) trigeminal neuralgia, compression of the 5th CN; (2) hemifacial spasm, compression of the 7th CN; (3) vestibulocochlear neuralgia, compression of the 8th CN; and (4) glossopharyngeal neuralgia, compression of the 9th CN.

Signs and Symptoms: Depends on which CN is affected, however, pain is the most common symptom.

Imaging Characteristics:

MRI
The pulse sequences listed below in combination are helpful in detecting NVCS.

- 3D T2-weighted imaging.
- 3D TOF-MRA.
- 3D T1-weighted imaging.
- Diffusion tensor imaging (DTI) with tractography.

Treatment: In most patients with classic trigeminal neuralgia, microvascular decompression (MVD) surgery produces immediate relief of symptoms. Separating the cranial nerve from the blood vessel may also be accomplished by using soft material such as Teflon to reduce the irritation. Ablative procedures, which may injure a portion of the cranial nerve, may be accomplished using stereotactic radiosurgery. Of all these procedures, MVD is the most durable and has the lowest risk of sensory deficits.

Prognosis: Good.

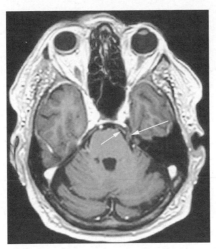

FIGURE 1. **Neurovascular Compression Syndrome.** MRA-TOF shows contact between the left posterior cerebral artery (PCA) (*short arrow*) and the left trigeminal nerve CN 5 (*long arrow*). In this individual, the vascular loop induced trigeminal neuralgia.

Superior Sagittal Sinus Thrombosis

Description: A thrombus is a blockage of the cerebral venous sinus. The superior sagittal sinus (SSS) is most commonly affected followed by the transverse and sigmoid sinuses, cerebral vein, straight vein, and cerebellar veins.

Etiology: Risk factors for SSS thrombosis may be associated with trauma, tumor compression, infection, oral contraceptive use, pregnancy, and idiopathic.

Epidemiology: A thrombosis is most commonly seen in the SSS. Tends to be seen in the second and third decade of life. Females are slightly more affected than males.

Signs and Symptoms: Headaches, seizures, and possible cerebral infarct.

Imaging Characteristics:

CT
- May show signs of an infarct.
- CT angiography (short delay following IV contrast injection of about 60 seconds) may be helpful in evaluating the cerebral venous sinus system.
- Shows venous filling defect.

MRI
- MR venography is best to demonstrate a filling defect in the SSS.
- Diffusion-weighted imaging is good to detect infarct.
- Loss of signal on time of flight (TOF) images.
- Conventional angiography should be considered if MR is not diagnostic.

Treatment: Anticoagulation therapy.

Prognosis: Depending on the extent of complications, there is a chance of death, especially in individuals who experienced coma, change in their mental status, intracerebral hemorrhage, and infection. For the vast majority of patients who do not experience any of the above-listed complications, their outlook is favorable with a full recovery.

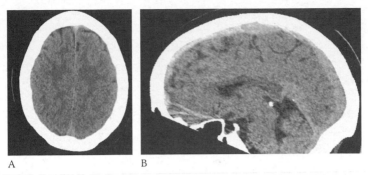

FIGURE 1. Superior Sagittal Sinus Thrombosis. Axial (A) and sagittal (B) NECTs show the anterior aspect of the superior sagittal sinus to be hyperdense.

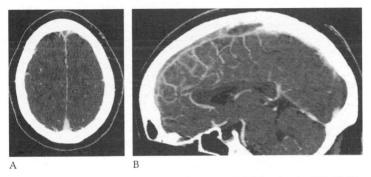

FIGURE 2. Superior Sagittal Sinus Thrombosis. Axial (A) and sagittal (B) CECT venogram shows a filling defect in the anterior superior sagittal sinus. The axial image demonstrates the "empty delta" sign. The sagittal image shows congestion of the cerebral veins that normally drain into superior sagittal sinus.

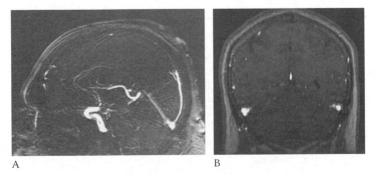

FIGURE 3. Superior Sagittal Sinus Thrombosis. MR venography shows lack of signal intensity in the superior sagittal sinus on the sagittal (A) and coronal (B) images.

BRAIN

DEGENERATIVE DISEASE

Alzheimer's Disease

Description: Alzheimer's disease (AD) is the most common dementing disorder affecting the elderly population.

Etiology: Factors such as atrophying of the hippocampal area, genetics, brain infarcts, and traumatic head injury are associated with the likelihood of having AD.

Epidemiology: The prevalence for AD is less than 1% before the age of 65; however, this quickly increases to 10% of the population over the age of 65 and between 30% and 50% over the age of 85 years and older. There seems to be a higher prevalence in women than in men.

Signs and Symptoms: Patients with AD present with a multifaceted loss of intellectual abilities such as memory, judgment, abstract thought and other higher cortical functions, and changes in personality and behavior.

Imaging Characteristics:

MRI and CT
- Primarily used to rule out other causes of dementia such as normal pressure hydrocephalus (NPH).
- CT used only when MRI is contraindicated.
- Diffuse cortical atrophy, usually more prominent in the temporal lobes.
- Hippocampal atrophy may be seen.
- Increases in ventricular size, sulcal size, Sylvian size, and total CSF volume are seen.
- MR spectroscopy (MRS) shows reduced levels of N-acetyl aspartate (NAA) and increased levels of myoinositol.

Treatment: There is no treatment currently available to stop or slow the deterioration of brain cells.

Prognosis: Poor; with an 8- to 10-year survival.

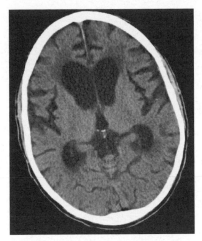

FIGURE 1. Alzheimer's Disease. Axial NECT shows diffuse cerebral atrophy with compensatory ventricular dilatation more than expected for the patient's age.

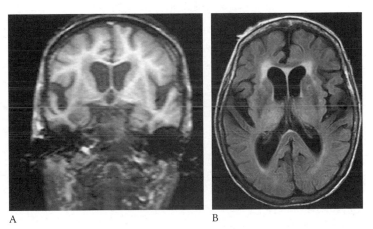

A   B

FIGURE 2. Alzheimer's Disease. Coronal T1W (A) and axial FLAIR (B) images show temporal-parietal atrophy and ventricular enlargement. The increased signal in the periventricular white matter on the FLAIR image is due to chronic small vessel ischemic change.

Multi-Infarct Dementia

Description: Multi-infarct dementia (MID) is the second most common form of dementia (following Alzheimer disease) in people older than 65 years of age. MID may also be called vascular dementia.

Etiology: Usually occurs as a result of a series of small strokes.

Epidemiology: Affects approximately 40 per 100,000 population. Estimates of 10% to 20% of all forms of dementia are MID. Incidences of MID are higher in males than in females. Individuals with African descent have a higher incidence than white people.

Signs and Symptoms:
- Difficulty in performing simple tasks.
- Language difficulty such as recalling familiar objects.
- Confusion, forgetfulness.
- Personality change.
- Depression, agitation, and delusions.
- Withdrawal from social contact.

Imaging Characteristics: MRI is more sensitive than CT and is the imaging modality of choice.

CT
- Multiple cortical and subcortical lacunar infarcts.

MRI
- Multiple cortical and subcortical lacunar infarcts.
- Decreased signal intensity of white matter on T1-weighted images.
- T2-weighted and FLAIR images show multiple hyperintense ischemic foci in the white matter.

Treatment: Treatment for MID is symptomatic.

Prognosis: Poor.

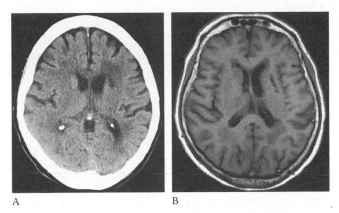

A   B

FIGURE 1. Multi-Infarct Dementia. Axial NECT (A) and T1W (B) images show confluent periventricular low-attenuation white matter changes and an old infarct involving the left subinsular region.

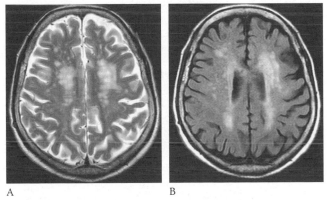

A   B

FIGURE 2. Multi-Infarct Dementia. Axial T2W (A) and axial FLAIR (B) images show extensive confluent periventricular white matter hyperintensity from prior infarcts as well as diffuse cerebral atrophy.

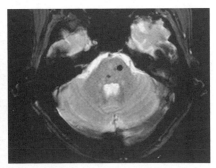

FIGURE 3. Multi-Infarct Dementia. Proton density (PD)-weighted axial image shows two small areas of very low signal (susceptibility artifact) in the pons from prior hemorrhage.

Normal-Pressure Hydrocephalus

Description: Normal-pressure hydrocephalus (NPH) is an idiopathic type of communicating hydrocephalus.

Etiology: Idiopathic.

Epidemiology: Tends to occur in the elderly (>65 years of age).

Signs and Symptoms: NPH is described by a triad of clinical characteristics which consists of dementia, gait disturbance, and urinary incontinence.

Imaging Characteristics:

CT and MRI
- Dilation of the ventricular system.
- Sulcal dilation.
- Dilation of the Sylvian fissure.
- Diffusion tensor imaging (DTI) is helpful in identifying small changes in periventricular white matter structures in the corpus callosum and corticospinal motor tract.

Treatment: Following ventriculoperitoneal (VP) shunting, patients may experience an improvement in their gait, urinary control, and cognitive ability.

Prognosis: If untreated, this condition will worsen. Early diagnosis and treatment increase the chance of a good recovery.

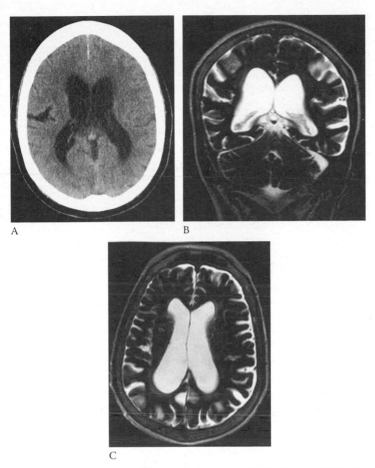

FIGURE 1. **Normal-Pressure Hydrocephalus.** Axial NECT (A), coronal T2W (B), and axial T2W (C) images show ventriculomegaly with rounding of the frontal horns which is out of proportion to the sulcal enlargement.

Parkinson's Disease

Description: Parkinson's disease (PD) is a neurodegenerative disorder characterized by progressive dementia, bradykinesia, shuffling gait, rigidity, and involuntary tremors.

Etiology: Unknown; however, genetic and environmental influences are suspected to be involved.

Epidemiology: Approximately 1% of the population over 50 years of age is affected. There is a genetic tendency in about 5% to 10% of those affected with PD.

Signs and Symptoms: Symptoms typically appear between 40 and 70 years of age. There are three characteristic signs: tremors, rigidity, and slowness in movement (bradykinesia).

Imaging Characteristics:

CT
- Shows nonspecific atrophy with enlarged ventricles and sulci.

MRI
- T2-weighted images show narrowing of the substantia nigra.
- MRS shows decrease in N-acetylaspartate (NAA) and a significant increase in the ratio of lactate to NAA.
- Ring-enhancing focus with vasogenic edema is typically seen about 3 months post-radiosurgery.

Treatment: Treatment is focused on controlling the symptoms. New treatments focusing on image-guided stereotactic approaches include (1) ablative procedures (thalamotomy, pallidotomy, and subthalamotomy); (2) deep brain stimulation (DBS); (3) restore degenerated tissue with brain grafting; and (4) gamma-knife radiosurgery.

Prognosis: Though PD is not fatal, it does reduce the life span of the patient.

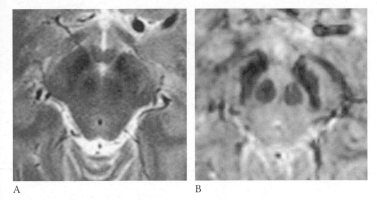

A   B

FIGURE 1. Parkinson's Disease. Axial T2W (A) and PD (B) images of the upper midbrain show thinning of the pars compacta (substantia nigra) as a narrowed hyperintense band of gray matter between the hypointense crural fibers anteriorly and red nuclei posteriorly.

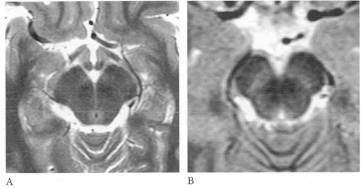

A   B

FIGURE 2. Parkinson's Disease. Axial T2W (A) and PD (B) images show normal thickness of the pars compacta.

BRAIN

DEMYELINATING

Multiple Sclerosis

Description: Multiple sclerosis (MS) is a demyelinating disease that is characterized by multiple inflammatory plaques of demyelination involving the white matter tracts of the central nervous system (brain and spine). This progressive disease is further characterized by the destruction of the lipid and protein layer called the myelin sheath that insulates the axon part of the nerve cell. The areas of demyelination are commonly referred to as "plaques." Multiple sclerosis may go through periods of exacerbation and remission.

Etiology: Unknown. However, theories suggest a slow-acting viral infection and an autoimmune response. Other theories suggest environmental and genetic factors.

Epidemiology: Females are slightly more affected than males at a ratio of 3:2. The incidence rate is between 18 and 50 years of age. In addition, MS is most commonly in people of European decent, less likely in Asians, and rarely in black Africans.

Signs and Symptoms: Patients may present with paresthesia, or abnormal sensations in the extremities or on one side of the face, numbness, tingling, or a "pins and needles" type of feeling, muscle weakness, vertigo, visual disturbances, such as nystagmus, diplopia (double vision), and partial blindness, extreme emotional changes, ataxia, abnormal reflexes, and difficulty in urinating.

Imaging Characteristics: MRI is the imaging modality of choice for diagnosis of MS.

MRI
- T1-weighted images appear isointense to hypointense.
- Proton density–weighted images appear hyperintense.
- T2-weighted images appear hyperintense.
- Active plaques may show contrast enhancement.

Treatment: There is no specific treatment for MS.

- Corticosteroids and other drugs, however, are used to treat the symptoms.
- Physical therapy may help postpone or prevent specific disabilities.

Prognosis: The course of the multiple sclerosis disease process is varied and unpredictable.

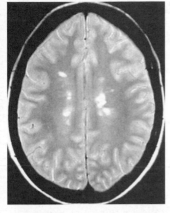

FIGURE 1. **Multiple Sclerosis.** MR proton density axial image shows ovoid hyperintense lesions (Dawson fingers) in the centrum semiovale bilaterally.

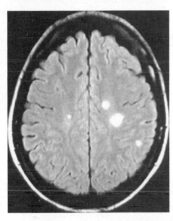

FIGURE 2. **Multiple Sclerosis.** Postcontrast T1-weighted axial MR shows enhancement of active multiple sclerosis plaques.

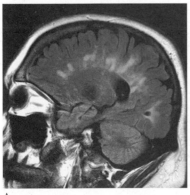

A   B

FIGURE 3. **Multiple Sclerosis.** Sagittal (A) and axial FLAIR (B) images show classic "Dawson fingers" as bilateral ovoid/linear hyperintense areas perpendicular to the callososeptal interface.

BRAIN
INFECTION

Brain Abscess

Description: Intracranial abscess is a free or encapsulated collection of pus that usually is located in the frontal, temporal, or parietal lobes of the brain.

Etiology: Usually occurs secondary to some other infection (e.g., otitis media, sinusitis, dental abscess, and mastoiditis). Other causes include subdural empyema, bacterial endocarditis, human immunodeficiency virus infection, bacteremia, pulmonary or pleural infection, abdominal/pelvic infections, and open head injuries.

Epidemiology: Males are twice as likely to be affected as females. Brain abscesses can occur at any age; however, the median age is between 30 and 40 years.

Signs and Symptoms: Patients may present with headaches, nausea and vomiting, change in mental status, afebrile or low-grade fever, seizures, and papilledema.

Imaging Characteristics:

CT
- Hypodense to isodense on noncontrast study.
- Ring-like enhancement with contrast.
- Marked edema appearance surrounding the abscess.

MRI
- Hypointense to gray matter on T1-weighted images.
- Hyperintense to gray matter on T2-weighted images with surrounding edema.
- Ring-like enhancement following administration of contrast.

Treatment: Antibiotics and possible surgical intervention are used in the treatment of brain abscesses.

Prognosis: A survival rate of 80% or greater when diagnosed early.

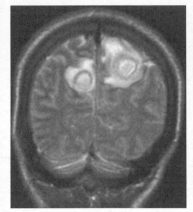

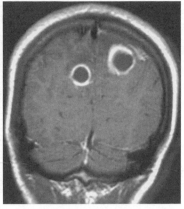

FIGURE 1. Brain Abscess. T2-weighted coronal image demonstrating round hyperintense lesions in bilateral occipital lobes with low-signal peripheral rim. There is moderate surrounding edema.

FIGURE 2. Brain Abscess. Postcontrast T1-weighted coronal image demonstrating ring-like contrast-enhancing lesions in the occipital lobes.

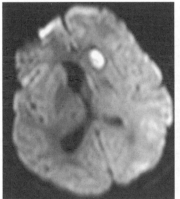

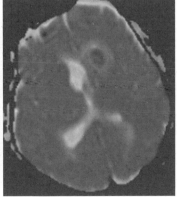

A

B

FIGURE 3. Brain Abscess. Axial DWI (A) shows high signal within the lesion and corresponding decreased signal on the ADC map (B) consistent with restricted diffusion commonly seen in an abscess.

Cysticercosis

Description: Cysticercosis is the most common parasitic infection of the central nervous system. Almost all cases of cysticercosis involve the brain.

Etiology: Results from the ingestion of ova of the pork tapeworm, *Taenia solium*.

Epidemiology: Most common CNS parasitic infection worldwide. Endemic in Mexico, Central and South America, Eastern Europe, Africa, and parts of Asia. Most cases in developed countries occur in immigrants from endemic areas. CNS involvement occurs in 60% to 90% of infected patients.

Signs and Symptoms: Seizures are most commonly seen in CNS involvement.

Imaging Characteristics:

CT
- Depicts spherical CSF-filled (hypodense) cysts.
- Ring-enhancing lesions on contrast studies.
- May show calcified lesions.

MRI
- The cyst appears hypointense on T1-weighted sequences.
- A scolex (the attachment organ of a tapeworm) may be seen in the center of the cyst on T1-weighted images.
- Ring-like enhancement of the cyst on T1-weighted contrast studies.
- Edema and the cyst appear hyperintense on T2-weighted images.

Treatment: An anthelmintic agent such as praziquantel or albendazole. These agents are used to kill the parasite. Surgical intervention may be required to remove intraventricular cysts, ventricular shunting, or both.

Prognosis: Morbidity usually results from dying larvae that bring about an intense inflammatory response.

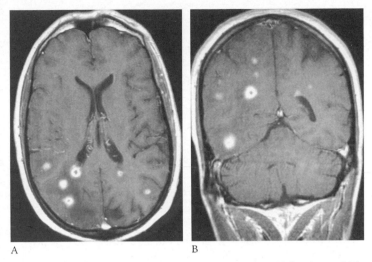

FIGURE 1. **Cysticercosis.** MRI postcontrast T1-weighted axial (A) and coronal (B) images demonstrate multiple small, round, enhancing lesions in the bilateral occipital lobes with surrounding low-signal edema.

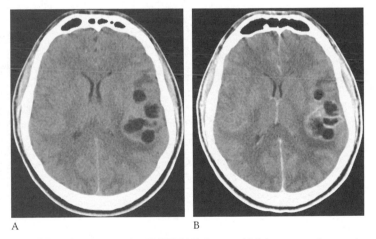

FIGURE 2. **Cysticercosis.** Axial NECT (A) shows multiple low-attenuation cysts in the subarachnoid space of the left Sylvian fissure. Axial postcontrast CT (B) shows rim enhancement of the cystic structures.

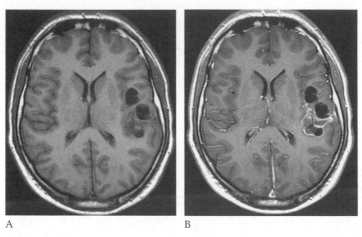

A   B

FIGURE 3. Cysticercosis. Pre- (A) and postcontrast (B) axial T1W images show similar findings to the CT (Figure 2).

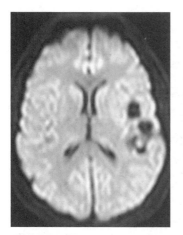

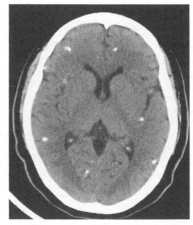

FIGURE 4. Cysticercosis. Axial DWI shows no restricted diffusion, differentiating it from an abscess which has restricted diffusion.

FIGURE 5. Cysticercosis. NECT shows multiple calcifications as a result of prior neurocysticercosis.

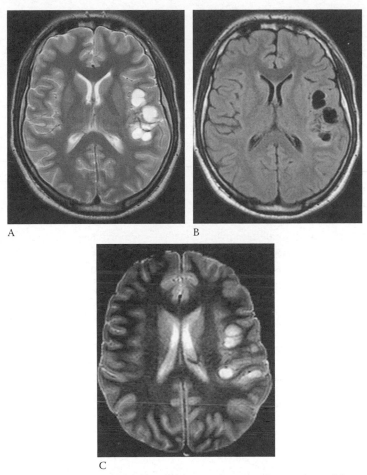

FIGURE 6. Cysticercosis. T2W axial (A) image shows that the central area of the cyst follows the CSF signal characteristics and is high intensity. Axial FLAIR (B) shows the CSF isointense to the CSF. There is mild hyperintense signal consistent with edema around the posterior cysts. T2 FFE (C) shows a small eccentric low signal within the cysts which may represent a small calcified scolex.

BRAIN
TRAUMA

Brain Herniation

Description: Brain herniation occurs when significant mass effect displaces the brain. Depending on the direction of the force created by the mass effect, five types of herniations may be seen.

- Subfalcine: Hemispheric mass effect shifts midline structures.
- Central transtentorial: Temporal mass effect pushes the temporal lobe (uncus) downward through the tentorium and compresses the oculomotor nerve (CN III), posterior cerebral artery, and midbrain which can result in small hemorrhages (Duret's hemorrhages) of the brainstem. Also called an uncal herniation.
- Tonsillar: Posterior fossa mass effect compresses the fourth ventricle. The cerebellar tonsils and cerebellum are forced down through the foramen magnum resulting in compression on the brainstem.
- Vermian: Superior cerebellar mass effect resulting in an upward herniation of the vermis and cerebellar tissue.
- Transalar: Central anterior mass effect results in a herniation of the frontal lobe over the greater wing of the sphenoid bone and backward movement of the Sylvian fissure, middle cerebral artery, and temporal lobe.

Etiology: Mass effect as result of head trauma, swelling, and mass lesion.

Epidemiology: The frequency of brain herniations depends largely on the etiology.

Signs and Symptoms: Level of consciousness (LOC), abnormal pupil and eye function, verbal and motor response (Glasgow Coma Scale), respiratory and cardiac arrest.

Imaging Characteristics:

MRI and CT
- Best seen on coronal images.
- Fractures, hemorrhage, and edema may be seen.
- Mass effect.
- Compression of the ipsilateral lateral ventricle.
- Dilatation of contralateral ventricle if foramen of Monro is obstructed.
- Midline shift of septum pellucidum.
- MR is best for seeing the tonsillar herniation with sagittal images.

Treatment: Treatments are designed to decrease the effects of intracranial pressure (ICP). Mannitol is used as a diuretic. Corticosteroids may help in reducing the effect of brain swelling and ICP. Shunting may be used to drain fluid such as blood. Surgery may be helpful in decompressing the brain.

Prognosis: Depends on the cause, duration, and degree of unconsciousness. Prognosis is usually poor with the possibility of brain death. A better prognosis may be seen in patients who have experienced a short time of unconsciousness.

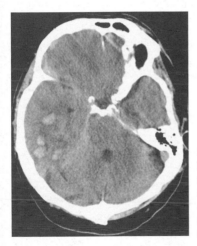

FIGURE 1. **Brain Herniation.** Axial NECT shows hyperdense blood in the right parietotemporal lobe with surrounding edema resulting in mass effect and with transtentorial (uncal) herniation demonstrated by obliteration of the suprasellar cistern.

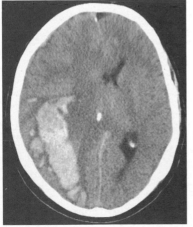

FIGURE 2. **Brain Herniation.** Axial NECT shows a large amount of hyperdense hemorrhagic blood in the right hemisphere with surrounding edema resulting in mass effect and a right-to-left midline shift with efface of the left lateral ventricle and subfalcine herniation.

Diffuse Axonal Injury

Description: Diffuse axonal injuries (DAI) occur when the axon of the neuron is injured (sheared) from a rapid deceleration.

Etiology: Results from a rapid deceleration such as in a high-speed motor vehicle accident.

Epidemiology: This injury can occur in anyone who experiences a high-speed rapid deceleration.

Signs and Symptoms: DAI is a severe injury to the brain and may be a closed head injury with an immediate loss of consciousness followed by a persistent vegetative state. Damage to the axons occurs at the time of the accident, and swelling occurs as a secondary factor.

Imaging Characteristics: MRI has more sensitivity than CT and is the imaging modality of choice.

CT
* May appear normal in 50% to 80% of cases except for diffuse cerebral edema.
* Small punctate "tissue tear" hemorrhages may be seen. These do not always indicate DAI.

MRI
* T1-weighted images appear isointense to surrounding tissue (non-hemorrhagic) and hyperintense (hemorrhagic).
* T2-weighted images appear hyperintense (nonhemorrhagic).
* Diffusion-weighted imaging is sensitive to seeing DAI as hyperintense.
* T2-weighted and FLAIR show DAI as hyperintense.
* Most DAI lesions are nonhemorrhagic.
* GRE images show (petechial hemorrhages) DAI as hypointense.

Treatment: Stabilizing and reducing brain swelling is the initial focus. Approximately 90% will remain in an unconscious vegetative state. The remaining 10% may regain consciousness with severe impairments. Various types of rehabilitation may be needed.

Prognosis: Mortality rate is 50%.

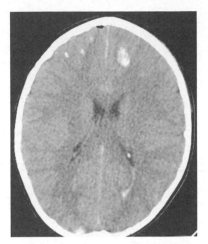

FIGURE 1. Diffuse Axonal Injury (DAI).
NECT shows a few small intraparenchymal
hyperdense foci of acute hemorrhage in the
frontal lobes and right posterior parietal lobe
due to "shear injury."

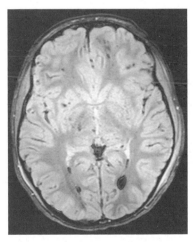

**FIGURE 2. Diffuse Axonal Injury
(DAI).** Axial gradient echo MR on the
same patient demonstrates the increased
sensitivity with MR. There are many
more punctate hypointense areas of
susceptibility artifact throughout the
cerebral hemispheres and basal ganglia from
small hemorrhagic shear injuries that were
not seen on CT.

Epidural Hematoma

Description: An epidural hematoma is a mass of blood frequently formed as a result of a trauma to the head. Though mostly arterial in origin, it is located between the skull and the dura mater in the temporoparietal region. Epidural hematomas are strongly associated with a linear skull fracture, which can cause a tear of the middle meningeal artery. Less common in occurrence are venous epidural hematomas which typically occur in the posterior fossa or adjacent to the occipital lobes of the cerebrum.

Etiology: Usually caused as a result of blunt trauma to the head with a tearing of the middle meningeal artery and blood then hemorrhaging into the epidural space.

Epidemiology: Individuals who have experienced blunt trauma to the head are at risk.

Signs and Symptoms: Patients may present with loss of consciousness (LOC), hemiparesis, headaches, dilated pupils, increased intracranial pressure (ICP), nausea and vomiting, dizziness, convulsions, and decerebrate rigidity.

Imaging Characteristics: Appears to be biconvex in shape and displacing the brain away from the skull. Noncontrast CT is the imaging modality of choice.

CT
- Underlying fracture.
- Acute stage hemorrhage will appear hyperdense.
- Subacute stage hemorrhage will appear isodense.
- Chronic stage may appear as hypodense.

MRI
- Subacute stage appears hyperintense on T1- and T2-weighted images.
- Acute stage hemorrhage will appear isointense on T1-weighted images and hypointense on T2-weighted images.

Treatment:
- Surgical emergency is required to remove the accumulated blood.

Prognosis: As a result of irreversible brain damage, mortality rates remain high even when diagnosed and treated early. However, if no complications arise, a normal recovery may occur. With early diagnosis and treatment prognosis is good; however, with large epidural hematomas, the outcome may result in neurologic deficit.

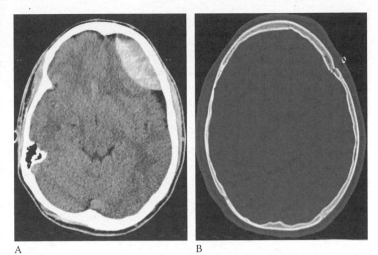

A   B

FIGURE 1. **Epidural Hematoma.** NECT (A) shows the typical biconvex hyperdense acute left frontal epidural hematoma resulting in mass effect on the left frontal lobe. NECT (B) of the same patient on bone windows shows an overlying left frontal skull fracture.

Subarachnoid Hemorrhage

Description: A subarachnoid hemorrhage (SAH) involves the escape of blood into the subarachnoid space especially the basal cisterns and into the cerebral spinal fluid (CSF) pathways.

Etiology: Subarachnoid hemorrhages occur most often as a result of a ruptured saccular (Berry) aneurysm. Other causes may include intracranial arteriovenous malformations (AVM), hypertension, or traumatic injury to the head.

Epidemiology: Approximately 11 out of every 100,000 people are affected annually. Traumatic incidents may occur at any age. The maximal incidence rate for a subarachnoid hemorrhage is in the fourth and fifth decade of life.

Signs and Symptoms: Headaches are the most common symptoms associated with SAH. Other complications may include loss of consciousness and focal neurologic deficits.

Imaging Characteristics: Noncontrast CT is the modality of choice for monitoring change of a subarachnoid hemorrhage.

CT
- Noncontrast examination reveals high-density acute blood present in the subarachnoid spaces (e.g., basilar cisterns and Sylvian fissures).

MRI
- MRI is not suitable for imaging most situations.
- FLAIR images have most sensitivity.
- FLAIR images show blood as hyperintensity in the subarachnoid space (CSF normally is nulled and therefore is not visible).
- MRA is useful to diagnose most large aneurysms (>5 mm).
- Conventional T1- and T2-weighted images are not very useful.
- Conventional angiography is the gold standard for the diagnosis of cerebral aneurysms.

Treatment: Treat the underlying aneurysm by placing a small metal clip or ligation around the neck of the aneurysm. Neuroradiologic intervention techniques available for treatment of intracranial aneurysms also include Guglielmi detachable coil (GD) coils. Prevent complications of a SAH (i.e., vasospasms, rebleeding, and hydrocephalus).

Prognosis: Varies depending on the severity of the initial hemorrhage and possibility of rebleeding and vasospasm.

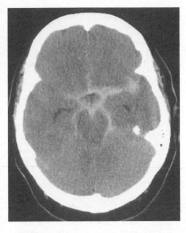

FIGURE 1. Subarachnoid Hemorrhage.
Noncontrast axial CT demonstrates blood in
the basilar cisterns as well as Sylvian fissures.

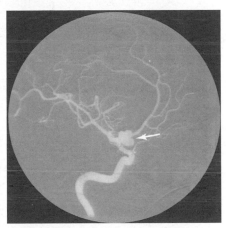

**FIGURE 2. Intracranial
Aneurysm.** Carotid arteriogram
demonstrates a large lobulated
aneurysm of the internal carotid
artery near its bifurcation.

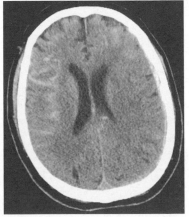

FIGURE 3. Subarachnoid Hemorrhage.
Axial NECT shows hyperdense blood
within the right Sylvian fissure.

Subdural Hematoma

Description: A subdural hematoma (SDH) is a collection of venous blood located between the dura mater and the arachnoid membrane (subdural space). A subdural hematoma usually develops as a result of the head hitting an immovable object. Though SDHs occur as a result of trauma, seldom are they associated with a skull fracture.

Etiology: SDHs are usually the result of the head striking an immovable object. High-speed acceleration- or deceleration-related head injuries could result in the tearing of the veins between the cerebral cortex and the dural veins. May also result from birth trauma or child abuse.

Epidemiology: Individuals who have experienced blunt trauma to the head are at risk. However, symptoms may not arise immediately. There are three time intervals between trauma and the onset of clinical symptoms. These time intervals vary from (1) 24 to 48 hours after injury is defined as acute; (2) between 48 hours and 2 weeks as subacute; and (3) 7 to 10 days as chronic.

Signs and Symptoms: Patients may present with headaches, a change in mental status, motor and sensory deficits, increased intercranial pressure, and possible deterioration of the neurologic status.

Characteristics: CT is the preferred modality for the diagnosis of acute SDH, whereas MRI is more sensitive for a subacute or chronic SDH. Subdural hematomas typically are crescentic shaped, conforming to the contour of the cranium's inner table. They may extend into the interhemispheric or tentorial subdural space.

CT
- Acute stage appears hyperdense.
- Subacute stage appears isodense.
- Chronic stage appears hypodense.

MRI
- Acute stage appears hypointense to isointense on T1-weighted images and hypointense on T2-weighted images.
- Subacute stage appears hyperintense on T1-weighted images and hypointense on T2-weighted images.
- Chronic stage appears with a higher signal (intermediate) than CSF on T1-weighted images and hyperintense on T2-weighted images.

Treatment: A subdural hematoma may be drained through a burr hole or require a craniotomy to drain the accumulated blood.

Prognosis: The mortality rates for acute and chronic subdural hematomas are greater than 50% and less than 10%, respectively. Most patients resume preoperative functional status. Outcome is highly dependent on the presurgical neurologic status.

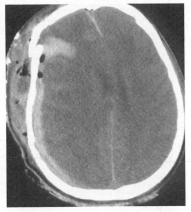

FIGURE 1. Subdural Hematoma. Noncontrast axial CT demonstrates a crescentic high-density acute right subdural hematoma in the right parietal and occipital region with mass effect on the right lateral ventricle and midline shift to the left. There is also a right frontal lobe hematoma (intracerebral). There is also a fracture of the right frontal bone as well as pneumocephalus.

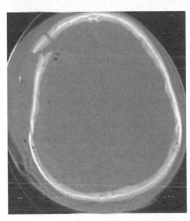

FIGURE 2. Skull Fracture. Bone window setting of an axial CT shows a skull fracture (right frontal bone). There is air (pneumocephalus) in the subdural space.

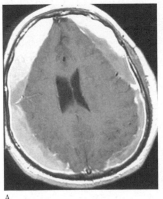
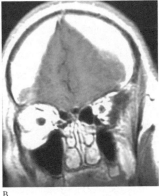

A   B

FIGURE 3. Subdural Hematoma. Noncontrast T1-weighted axial (A) and coronal (B) MR images demonstrate large bilateral, mostly high-signal, subacute subdural hematomas.

SPINE
CONGENITAL

Arnold-Chiari Malformation

Description: Arnold-Chiari malformations consist of a spectrum of congenital anomalies that affect the hindbrain. They are characterized by a downward elongation of the brainstem (medulla oblongata), cerebellum (cerebellar tonsils), and the fourth ventricle into the cervical portion of the spinal cord. Arnold-Chiari malformations are categorized into three types.

In an Arnold-Chiari Type I, the cerebellar tonsils alone are displaced 5 to 6 mm or more below the foramen magnum. There is no hydrocephalus involved and the fourth ventricle remains in its normal location. A syringohydromyelia (syrinx) of the cervical spinal cord may be seen. This may be associated with Klippel-Feil syndrome.

In an Arnold-Chiari Type II, the cerebellar tonsils and vermis of the fourth ventricle, cerebellum, and medulla oblongata have herniated down through the foramen magnum into the cervical spinal canal. Obstruction of the fourth ventricle results in hydrocephalus. This type is associated with myelomeningocele and agenesis of the corpus callosum.

An Arnold-Chiari Type III malformation is characterized by displacement of the cerebellum meninges, and sometimes the brainstem into an encephalocele. Encephaloceles result from a herniation of the brain or meninges, or both, through a skull defect. Characteristics seen in Type II Chiari malformations may be present. It occurs in approximately 1 in 4000 to 5000 deliveries.

Etiology: Though there are several theories of the cause of this malformation, the one that is generally accepted is that the posterior fossa is too small, causing a herniation of the brain stem and cerebellar tonsils through the foramen magnum into the upper cervical spinal canal.

Epidemiology: Type I Arnold-Chiari malformations are found more often in adults (incidentally by MRI) than in children. There does not seem to be any gender preference.

Signs and Symptoms: Hydrocephalus and developmental defects may be seen early on in infants. Young adults may be asymptomatic until neurologic deficits such as craniocervical junction abnormalities (e.g., progressive ataxia) occur.

Imaging Characteristics: MRI is the modality of choice for diagnosing this disorder.

CT

- The effectiveness of demonstrating this anomaly with CT is limited due to the bony surroundings and axial imaging.

MRI

- T1- and T2-weighted pulse sequences will demonstrate the downward herniation of the cerebellar tonsils through the foramen magnum into the upper cervical canal.
- Associated findings may include syringomyelia and hydrocephalus.

Treatment: Surgery intervention may be used to decompress the posterior fossa. Shunt placement is used to treat hydrocephalus.

Prognosis: Depends on the type, age of the patient when diagnosed, and extent of other related developmental defects. The prognosis for infants may be worse than for adults.

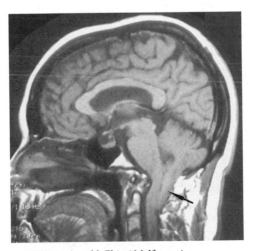

FIGURE 1. **Arnold-Chiari Malformation.**
T1-weighted sagittal image demonstrates downward herniation of the cerebellar tonsils (*arrow*) through the foramen magnum into the upper cervical spinal canal with compression of the medulla oblongata.

Syringomyelia/Hydromyelia

Description: Syringomyelia refers to any fluid-filled cavity within the spinal cord. A cavity in the cord may be due to central canal dilatation (hydromyelia) or a cavity eccentric to the central canal (syrinx). It is difficult to differentiate between these two entities.

Etiology: Approximately 50% of syringomyelias are congenital (Chiari malformation). Acquired cases are the result of intramedullary tumors, trauma, infarction, and hemorrhage. In some cases there is no known cause.

Epidemiology: Approximately 90% of syringomyelias occur in association with an Arnold-Chirai Type I malformation, but also may include, myelomeningocele, basilar skull impression (platybasia), atresia of the foramen of Magendie, or Dandy-Walker cysts.

Signs and Symptoms: Depends on the extent of the syrinx. The patient may experience sensory loss (loss of pain and temperature), muscle atrophy (lower neck, shoulders, arms, and hands), and thoracic scoliosis.

Imaging Characteristics: MRI is the modality of choice for the diagnosis of syringomyelia.

CT
♦ Postmyelogram CT demonstrates a contrast-filled syrinx surrounded by the hypodense spinal cord.

MRI
♦ Signal intensity of a syrinx may be isointense to CSF on T1-weighted images.
♦ Signal intensity of a syrinx would be isointense to CSF on T2-weighted images.

Treatment: Surgical drainage of the syrinx is the suggestive treatment.

Prognosis: Variable, depending on the extent of the syrinx.

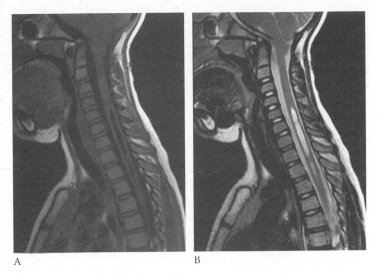

FIGURE 1. Syringomyelia. Sagittal T1W (A) shows abnormal low intramedullary signal and cord expansion. (B) The abnormal fluid within the spinal cord is hyperintense on the sagittal T2W image.

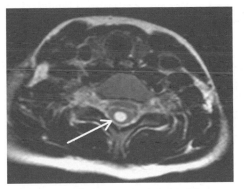

FIGURE 2. Syringomyelia. Axial T2W of the cervical spine shows hyperintense fluid in the spinal cord (*arrow*) consistent with a syrinx.

Tethered Cord

Description: A tethered cord is a condition in which the conus medullaris is prevented from ascending to its usual position at the level of L1-L2. It is tethered at an abnormally low position by a tight, short, thickened filum terminale, fibrous bands, intradural lipoma, or some other intradural abnormality.

Etiology and Epidemiology: This congenital abnormality is seen in neonates.

Signs and Symptoms: Patient presents with muscle weakness, abnormal lower limb reflexes, bowel and bladder dysfunction, back pain, and scoliosis.

Imaging Characteristics: MRI is the imaging modality of choice for the diagnosis of a tethered cord.

MRI
- Tip of the conus medullaris is below the level of L2.
- T1-weighted axial shows a thickened (>2 mm in diameter) filum terminale.
- The conus medullaris may be tethered by spina bifida occulta and/or intradural lipoma (posteriorly displaced by fat), glial cells, and collagen.

Treatment: Surgery in infancy or early childhood is required to prevent progressive neurologic deficit.

Prognosis: Depends on the extent of the tethered cord and the age of the young child at the time of diagnosis and treatment.

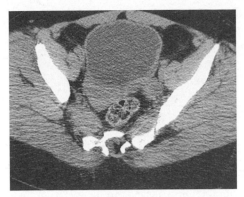

FIGURE 1. **Tethered Cord.** Axial contrasted CT scan through pelvis shows abnormal fat density within the sacral spinal canal consistent with terminal lipoma.

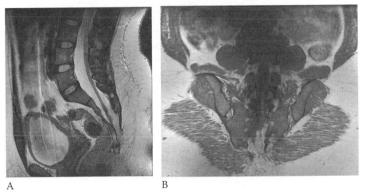

A   B

FIGURE 2. **Tethered Cord.** Sagittal T2W (A) and coronal oblique T1W (B) images through lumbar spine demonstrate thickened terminal filum and a terminal lipoma. Note: extension of fat through spinal dysraphism into spinal canal.

SPINE
DEGENERATIVE

Herniated Disk

Description: A herniated disk is also referred to as a ruptured or protruded disk. A herniated disk occurs when part or the entire nucleus pulposus (the soft, gelatinous, central portion of an intervertebral disk) is forced through the disk's weakened or torn outer ring (annulus fibrosus). This extruded herniated disk may impinge upon spinal nerve roots as they exit from the spinal canal or on the spinal cord itself.

Etiology: Herniated disks may result from severe trauma or strain, or may be related to intervertebral joint degeneration. In older patients with degenerative disk disease, minor trauma may cause herniation.

Epidemiology: About 90% of herniated disks occur in the lumbosacral spine, with the majority of these occurring at L5-S1, and the rest at either L4-L5 or L3-L4. A small percent of herniated disks involve the cervical spine, with the majority of these being at C5-C6 and C6-C7. Only 1% to 2% of herniated disks occur in the thoracic spine.

Signs and Symptoms: Patients with lumbosacral herniated disks will present with low back pain, radiating to the buttocks, legs, and feet, usually unilaterally. Sensory and motor loss, muscle weakness, and atrophy of the leg muscles may be experienced if a lumbar spinal nerve root is compressed. Cervical disk herniations present with pain in the neck and upper extremities and weakness, and neurologic deficits, such as muscle spasms, numbness, and tingling are common symptoms.

Imaging Characteristics: As a result of excellent soft tissue resolution and multiplanar imaging, MRI is the imaging modality of choice for diagnosing herniated disk.

MRI and CT
- Demonstrate disc degeneration.
- Herniated disc usually laterized to one side compressing the thecal sac and nerve root.
- Free disc fragments may migrate superiorly or inferiorly.

Treatment: Conservative treatment consists of bed rest, heat, exercise, and medication ranging from anti-inflammatory drugs to muscle relaxants. Patients not responding to conservative treatment may require surgical intervention.

Prognosis: Prognosis is very mixed, dependent on the severity of damage, the quality and skill of surgical intervention, the age, size, and weight of the patient, and whether there is a physically active or sedentary lifestyle.

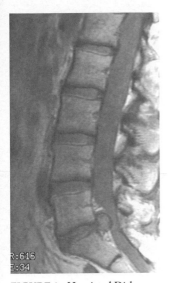

FIGURE 1. Herniated Disk.
T1-weighted sagittal MR image
shows herniated disc at the L5-S1
level.

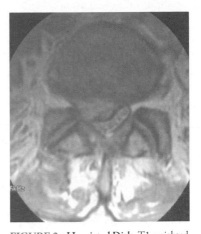

FIGURE 2. Herniated Disk. T1-weighted
axial MR image demonstrates right-sided
herniated disk at the L5-S1 level compressing
the right side of the thecal sac and nerve root.

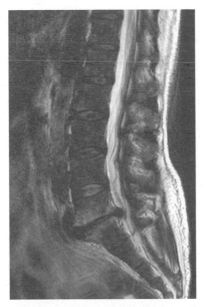

FIGURE 3. Herniated Disk. T2W sagittal
MR of L5-S1 verify disc bulge. End-plate
hyperintensity about this disc space was
degenerative.

Spinal Stenosis

Description: Spinal stenosis may be defined as the narrowing of the spinal canal and lateral recesses as a result of progressive degenerative disease of the disk, bone, and ligament. Problems arise when the spinal canal and cord is constricted. Mostly involves the cervical and lumbar spine.

Etiology: Spinal stenosis may be categorized as either congenital (developmental) or acquired. Congenital spinal stenosis may be due to achondroplasia or anomaly, or may be idiopathic. Acquired central spinal stenosis may result from several manifestations including degenerative disk disease, ligamentum flavum hypertrophy, spondylolisthesis, bulging disk, and trauma.

Epidemiology: Most commonly found in the cervical and lumbar spine.

Signs and Symptoms: When the cervical portion of the spine is involved, the patient may present with a radiculopathy, myelopathy, or neck or shoulder pain. If the lumbar spine is affected, the patient may present with a limping type of gait (neurogenic or spinal claudication), low back pain, or paresthesia of the lower extremities.

Imaging Characteristics: MRI is the modality of choice for diagnosing spinal stenosis. CT following myelography would be the next best choice for imaging spinal stenosis.

MRI and CT
- Narrowing of the spinal canal, lateral recess, and neural foramen.
- Bulging discs.
- Hypertrophy of facet joints and ligamentum flavum.
- Spondylolisthesis.
- Compression of the thecal sac and nerve roots.

Treatment: Surgical intervention may be considered.

Prognosis: This condition is progressive.

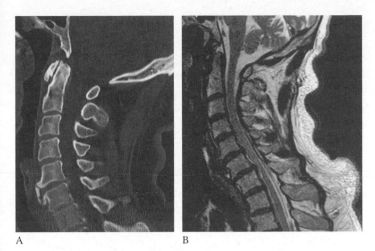

A   B

FIGURE 1. Spinal Stenosis. Sagittal CT (A) and T2 MR (B) images through the cervical spine demonstrate multilevel disc bulges most notable at C5-C7, causing moderate canal stenosis.

Spondylolisthesis

Description: Spondylolisthesis is the displacement or slippage, either anterior or posterior, of a vertebra over an inferior vertebra (usually the fifth lumbar vertebra over the sacrum, or the fourth lumbar vertebra over the fifth), causing a misalignment of the vertebral column. Type I involves a 25% vertebral displacement over the vertebra that is immediately inferior to it, Type II a 50% vertebral displacement, and Type III a 75% vertebral displacement over the inferior vertebra. Type IV involves anything over a 75% vertebral displacement over the inferior vertebra.

Etiology: Spondylolisthesis may result from acute trauma, congenital or acquired fibrous defects in the pars interarticularis (spondylolysis), or as a result of spinal instability due to degenerative changes involving the disk and facet joints.

Epidemiology: Spondylolisthesis occurs in 60% of patients with spondylolysis, which occurs in approximately 5% of the population. The L5-S1 interspace accounts for 90% of the cases of spondylolisthesis, with the majority of those cases being anterior displacement of the L5 vertebra. The L4-L5 interspace accounts for approximately 10% of spondylolisthesis cases, with most involving anterior slippage of L4 vertebra. Cervical spondylolisthesis comprises less than 1% of all cases.

Signs and Symptoms: Patients may present with low back pain and/or stiffness and loss of function. Tight hamstrings may force the patient to walk with the knees bent and a short stride, causing poor posture or unusual gait.

Imaging Characteristics: Plain films are usually sufficient to make the diagnosis.

CT
- Sagittal reformatted images demonstrate a shifting of a vertebra over an inferior vertebra.
- Shows pars interarticularis defects (spondylolysis).

MRI
- Shows forward slippage of one vertebra over another. Best seen on a sagittal image.
- Shows other associated findings (e.g., degenerative disk disease and spinal stenosis).

Treatment: Conservative treatment is usually initiated to treat the patient's symptoms. Surgery may be indicated in symptomatic patients who do not respond to conservative treatment.

Prognosis: May vary depending on the type and other associated findings.

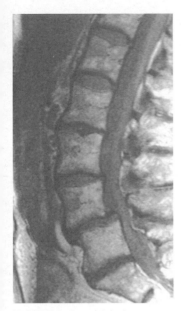

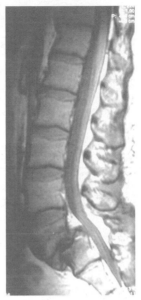

FIGURE 1. Spondylolisthesis Grade I. Sagittal T1-weighted MR image of the lumbar spine demonstrates mild forward displacement of the L4 vertebral body over L5. This is consistent with grade I spondylolisthesis. Degenerative changes of L4-L5 and L5-S1 discs noted.

FIGURE 2. Spondylolisthesis Grade II. T1-weighted sagittal image demonstrates a forward displacement of the L5 vertebral body over S1 consistent with a grade II spondylolisthesis. Note: The degenerative changes of the L5/S1 disk.

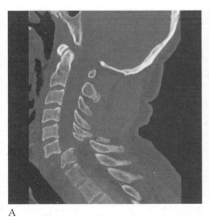

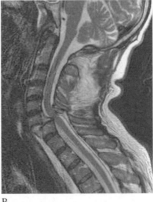

A   B

FIGURE 3. Spondylolisthesis. Sagittal CT (A) demonstrates traumatic (Type 4) anterolisthesis of C6 on C7 with bilateral jumped facets (not shown). Sagittal T2W MR (B) shows anterolisthesis and extensive ligamentous/soft tissue injury.

SPINE

DEMYELINATING

Multiple Sclerosis (Spinal Cord)

Description: Multiple sclerosis (MS) is a demyelinating disease affecting the spinal cord (see the section "Brain, Multiple Sclerosis"). The areas of demyelination are commonly referred to as "plaques." Multiple sclerosis may go through periods of exacerbation and remission.

Etiology: The exact cause of multiple sclerosis is unknown; however, theories suggest a slow-acting viral infection and an autoimmune response. Other theories suggest environmental and genetic factors.

Epidemiology: Multiple sclerosis commonly involves the spinal cord. Rarely is MS seen in children and older adults. Females are slightly more affected than males.

Signs and Symptoms: Patient presents with focal neurologic attacks, progressive deterioration, and ultimately permanent neurologic dysfunction. Other complications include sensory and motor dysfunction.

Imaging Characteristics: MRI is the imaging modality of choice for the diagnosis of multiple sclerosis in the spinal cord.

MRI
- T1-weighted images are useful to evaluate the spinal cord morphology.
- T2-weighted images demonstrate the MS plaque as high signal.
- Postcontrast T1-weighted images demonstrate enhancement of active MS plaques.
- FLAIR images improve MS plaque detection by suppressing CSF signal near the spinal cord.

Treatment: There is no specific treatment for MS.

- Corticosteroids and other drugs, however, are used to treat the symptoms.
- Physical therapy may help to postpone or prevent specific disabilities.

Prognosis: The course of the multiple sclerosis disease process is varied and unpredictable.

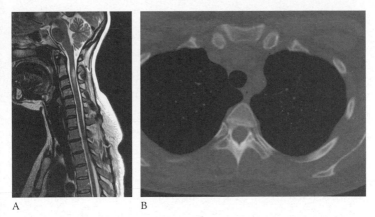

A   B

FIGURE 1. **Multiple Sclerosis (Spinal Cord).** Sagittal T2 MR (A) image through cervical spine demonstrates a well-delineated hyperintense lesion in this patient with known MS. Axial CT scan (B) at the level of the lesion shows no identifiable abnormality at that level.

SPINE
INFECTION

Vertebral Osteomyelitis

Description: Osteomyelitis is an inflammation of the bone caused by an infecting organism. It may be localized or spread through the bone to involve the marrow, cortex, periosteum, and soft tissue surrounding the affected area. Vertebral osteomyelitis usually occurs as a result of disk space infection; however, osteomyelitis may occur through hematogenous dissemination directly to the vertebral body. Pyogenic infections to the disk space are usually caused by a blood-borne pathogen from the lung or urinary tract. These pathogens get lodged in the region of the end-plate of the bone and destroy the disk space and the adjacent vertebral bodies.

Etiology: The majority (90%) of all bone and joint infections are caused by the *Staphylococcus aureus* microorganism and may occur following trauma or surgery. Other common microorganisms include *Escherichia coli* and *Proteus*.

Epidemiology: Osteomyelitis can occur in any location and patients at any age. Patients who are particularly vulnerable include diabetics, steroid users who are immunosuppressed, those on hemodialysis, and drug addicts, particularly heroin.

Signs and Symptoms: Patient presents with fever, malaise, pain, and swelling over the affected area.

Imaging Characteristics: MRI is the preferred imaging modality. A gallium scan or indium-111-labeled leukocyte scan can also be helpful.

MRI
- T1-weighted images show low-signal intensity.
- T2-weighted images show high-signal intensity.
- Postcontrast, fat-suppressed, T1-weighted images show enhancement in bone due to abscess formation and juxtacortical soft tissue enhancement.

Treatment: Antibiotic treatment is required. Severe cases may also need surgery.

Prognosis: Generally good, with early diagnosis and effective treatment.

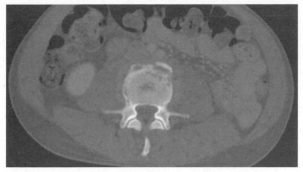

FIGURE 1. **Vertebral Osteomyelitis.** Axial (bone window) CT scan shows lytic destruction of the L4 vertebral body with abnormal enhancement involving the adjacent psoas muscles.

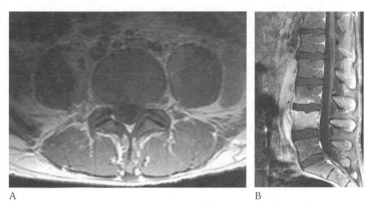

A   B

FIGURE 2. **Vertebral Osteomyelitis.** Postcontrast T1W fat-saturated axial (A) and sagittal (B) images through the lumbar spine demonstrate abnormal enhancement of L3 and L4 with extension into the psoas muscles bilaterally. Note: Right psoas muscle abscess.

SPINE
TUMOR

Metastatic Disease to the Spine

Description: Metastatic tumors involving the bony vertebrae of the spine. These tumors are, commonly, a devastating complication of disseminated cancer.

Etiology: Metastatic spread of a cancer from a primary tumor. Metastases to the spine occur primarily as the result of hematogenous spread.

Epidemiology: Any malignant tumor can involve the vertebral spine; however, breast carcinoma and lung carcinoma are the most common. Approximately 20% to 35% of all cancer patients may develop symptoms associated with metastasis to the vertebral spine. About 5% of affected patients develop symptoms related to spinal cord compression due to the collapse of one or more vertebrae, or epidural tumor spread. The thoracic (70%) and lumbar (20%) regions are most commonly affected with 10% involving the cervical regions. There is a propensity for colon carcinoma to spread to the lumbosacral spine and breast, and lung carcinoma to metastasis to the thoracic spine.

Signs and Symptoms: Patient with known cancer history presents with back pain and possible loss of sensory and motor function. Suspected spinal cord compression requires emergent neurosurgical evaluation.

Imaging Characteristics: Plain x-rays and nuclear medicine bone scan, CT, and MRI are useful imaging modalities.

CT
- CT is good for the evaluation of bone destruction.
- Shows osteolytic or osteoblastic bony metastatic lesion.

MRI
- MRI is excellent for the evaluation of spinal cord compression.
- T1-weighted images appear with low-signal intensity in the affected bony vertebrae.
- T2-weighted images appear with variable signal intensity in the affected bony vertebrae.
- Shows extension of the tumor into the spinal canal and spinal cord compression.

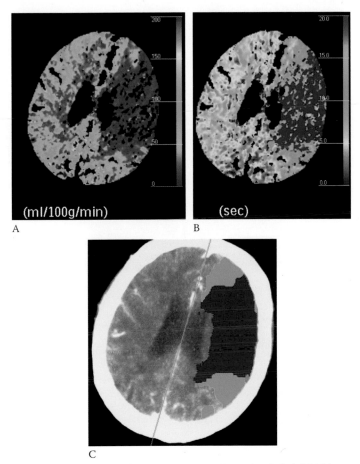

FIGURE 4. Ischemic Stroke. Same patient as in Figure 5 with the left MCA stroke. Shows decreased cerebral perfusion to this area (blue) (A). Mean transit time is prolonged (blue) (B). In image (C) red represents an infarct; green represents the penumbra of threatened (at risk) ischemic brain that may potentially be saved with an intervention.

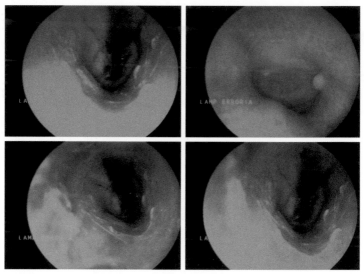

FIGURE 6. Glomus Tumor (Glomus Tympanicum). Clinical otoscopic images show a (blue) vascular mass located behind the eardrum. This corresponds to the mass seen on the cochlear promontory (Figure 3).

Treatment: Radiation therapy or surgery depending on the type of tumor. Spinal cord compression requires emergent radiation therapy or neurosurgery to prevent permanent paralysis.

Prognosis: A poor prognosis is expected for metastatic cancer.

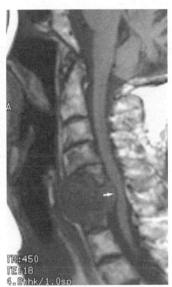

FIGURE 1. Spinal Metastasis.
T1-weighted sagittal image shows a large low-signal intensity lesion involving the C5-C6 vertebral bodies with encroachment of the anterior spinal canal and compression of the spinal cord (*arrow*).

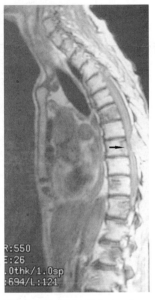

FIGURE 2. Spinal Metastasis.
T1-weighted image shows low-signal intensity lesions (*arrow*) of multiple vertebrae. There is marked compression of the spinal cord at the level of T8 (*arrow*).

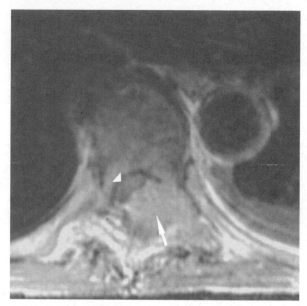

FIGURE 3. Spinal Metastasis. T1-weighted axial image shows a high-signal-intensity mass (*arrow*) encroaching on the spinal canal and compressing the spinal cord (*arrowhead*).

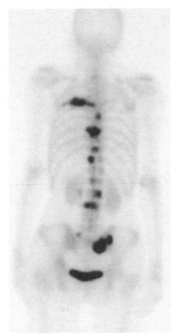

FIGURE 4. Spinal Metastasis.
Whole body bone scan shows multiple
areas of increased uptake involving the
thoracic and lumbar spine as well as the
left pelvis and right upper ribs.

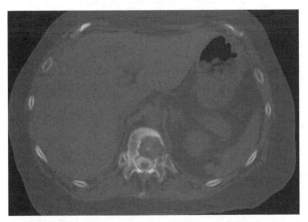

FIGURE 5. Spinal Metastasis. CT myelogram (bone window)
shows a lytic lesion in the lower thoracic vertebral body. Biopsy revealed
metastatic cancer.

Spinal Ependymoma

Description: A spinal ependymoma is the most common tumor of the spinal cord. They are benign and slow growing, and arise from the ependymal cells lining the central canal or from ependymal rests.

Etiology: These tumors develop from ependymal cells lining the central canal or from ependymal rests.

Epidemiology: Males are slightly more affected than females. The peak incidence is in the fourth and fifth decade of life. The majority of all spinal ependymomas occur in the lumbosacral region.

Signs and Symptoms: Patients most commonly present with pain. Some patients may complain of leg weakness and sphincter dysfunction.

Imaging Characteristics: MRI is the imaging modality of choice for the diagnosis of spinal ependymoma.

MRI
- Hypointense to isointense to the spinal cord on T1-weighted images.
- T2-weighted images produce a bright signal in the CSF and obscure the high signal of the tumor.
- Postcontrast T1-weighted image shows a homogeneous, well-circumscribed, high-signal tumor.

Treatment: Complete surgical resection.

Prognosis: A complete resection of the tumor usually results in a cure.

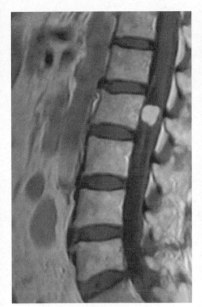

FIGURE 1. Spinal Ependymoma.
Postcontrast T1-weighted sagittal MR image demonstrates a round enhancing mass of the conus medullaris at the level of L2 consistent with an ependymoma.

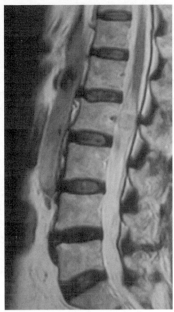

FIGURE 2. Spinal Ependymoma.
T2-weighted sagittal MR image demonstrates a 1.3-cm round mass with intermediate signal in the conus medullaris at the level of L2.

Spinal Hemangioma

Description: A vertebral hemangioma is the most common benign lesion incidentally found. Hemangiomas are slow-growing vascular tumors that generally do not cause symptoms. These lesions rarely result in compression or expansion of the vertebral body with subsequent cord compression.

Etiology: Unknown.

Epidemiology: Vertebral hemangiomas are the most common benign lesion of the spine and are present in more than 10% of all patients. Females are more affected than males by a ratio of 2:1. These lesions are most commonly located in the thoracic spine.

Signs and Symptoms: Nonspecific; these lesions are incidentally found.

Imaging Characteristics:

CT
- Bony striations associated with course, thickened trabeculae giving a "corduroy" appearance.
- Appear as low-attenuation (hypodense) area.

MRI
- T1-weighted images will appear hyperintense due to the presences of fat or hemorrhage.
- T2-weighted images will appear hyperintense.

Treatment: Symptomatic treatment.

Prognosis: Excellent; a hemangioma is a benign tumor.

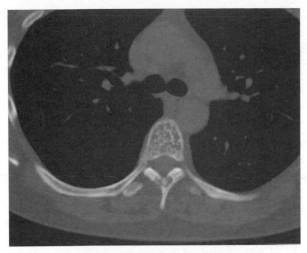

FIGURE 1. Spinal Hemangioma. Axial CT (bone window) shows classic striated pattern with thickened trabecula in a thoracic vertebral body.

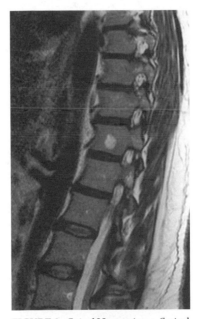

FIGURE 2. Spinal Hemangioma. Sagittal T2W MR image demonstrates hyperintense portion of thoracic vertebral body. Lesion appeared similarly hyperintense on T1 images, also consistent with hemangioma.

Spinal Meningioma

Description: Spinal meningiomas are benign and account for approximately 25% of all intradural tumors. They are characteristically hard, slow growing, and usually highly vascular.

Etiology: Meningiomas of the spine are believed to arise from the arachnoid cells located near the dorsal nerve root ganglia.

Epidemiology: Meningiomas of the spine occur much less frequently than intracranial meningiomas. Spinal meningiomas usually present after the fourth decade of life and occur more commonly in females than males. They are found most commonly in the thoracic region (80%), followed by the cervical region (17%), and least often in the lumbar region (3%).

Signs and Symptoms: Patient presents with pain associated with compression of the spinal cord and adjacent nerve roots. Sensory and motor dysfunctions such as weakness, bowel and bladder dysfunction, and paresthesias may be present.

Imaging Characteristics: MRI is the imaging modality of choice for the diagnosis of spinal meningioma.

CT
- Shows calcified meningiomas.
- CT myelography may demonstrate a blockage by an intradural/extramedullay mass.

MRI
- T1-weighted images are typically isointense to the spinal cord.
- T2-weighted images may present with either low-signal or high-signal intensity.
- Contrast-enhanced T1-weighted images show a homogeneous enhancing high-signal intensity mass.

Treatment: Complete surgical removal.

Prognosis: Good, this is a benign tumor.

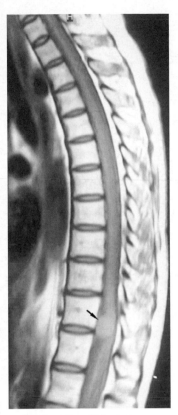

FIGURE 1. Spinal Meningioma.
T1-weighted sagittal image shows a
round isointense mass (*arrow*) at the
level of T6-T7.

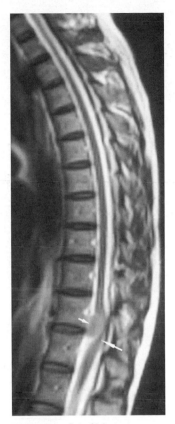

FIGURE 2. Spinal Meningioma.
T2-weighted sagittal image shows a
slightly high-signal intensity mass (*short
arrow*) at the level of T6-T7 displacing
the cord (*long arrow*) posteriorly.

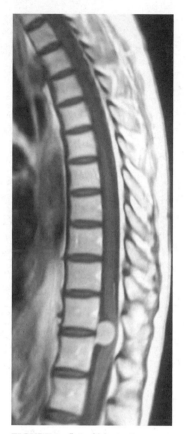

FIGURE 3. Spinal Meningioma.
Postcontrast T1-weighted sagittal
image shows intense homogeneous
enhancement of the mass at the level
of T6-T7.

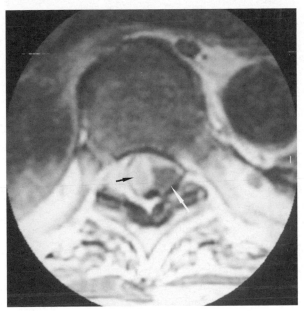

FIGURE 4. Spinal Meningioma. Postcontrast T1-weighted axial image shows a contrast-enhancing extramedullary mass in the right side of the spinal canal (*short arrow*) at T6-T7 with displacement of the cord (*long arrow*) to the left.

SPINE

TRAUMA

Burst Fracture

Description: A vertically oriented fracture of the vertebral body with lateral dispersion of the fracture fragments, usually with associated fractures in the posterior elements of the vertebra (e.g., lamina and/or spinous process).

Etiology: Usually the result of a flexion or axial loading traumatic force, causing a flexion-compression injury.

Epidemiology: Most commonly occurs between 16 and 25 years of age. Males are more affected than females.

Signs and Symptoms: Patient presents with low back pain, possibly extending down the buttocks and backs of legs. Neurologic deficits, such as numbness and/or tingling in the lower extremities, leg weakness, or paralysis may be present.

Imaging Characteristics: CT is the imaging modality to demonstrate bony anatomy, while MRI is better for showing soft tissue structures.

CT
- Fractures of vertebral body.
- Fractures of the pedicles and lamina.
- Shows displaced fracture fragments that may compromise the spinal canal.

MRI
- Excellent modality to evaluate the status of the spinal canal and spinal cord.
- May show cord hemorrhage.
- May show compromise of the spinal canal and compression of the spinal cord.
- May show associated ligamentous injury or herniated disk.

Treatment: Surgical stabilization of the damaged bone or vertebra via fusing or metallic bracing may be required.

Prognosis: Mixed and varied, dependent on the degree of damage and neurologic involvement of spinal nerve roots and spinal cord.

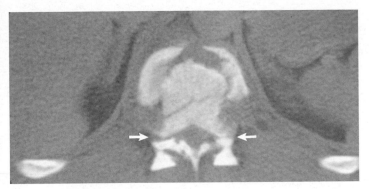

FIGURE 1. Comminuted Burst Fracture. Axial CT shows a burst fracture of T12 with displacement of the fracture fragment resulting in compromise of the spinal canal. Note: Fractures of the bilateral pedicles and associated small paraspinal hematoma (*arrows*).

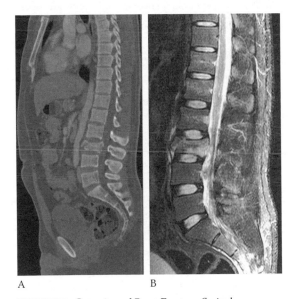

A   B

FIGURE 2. Comminuted Burst Fracture. Sagittal multiplanar reconstruction (MPR) CT (A) and sagittal T2W MR (B) images through the lumbar spine demonstrate a burst fracture of L3 with retropulsion of fragments. Note: Associated epidural hematoma.

C1 Fracture

Description: Three primary types of fractures have been identified involving the C1 vertebrae: (1) the posterior arch fracture usually occurs at the junction of the posterior arch and the lateral mass; (2) the lateral mass fracture usually occurs unilaterally with the fracture line passing either through the articular surface or just anterior and posterior to the lateral mass on one side; and (3) the burst fracture (Jefferson fracture) is characterized by four fractures, two in the anterior arch and two in the posterior arch. This fracture may present as a stable nondisplaced fracture with no encroachment on the spinal cord or as a displaced fracture with varying degrees of encroachment on the spinal cord. A displaced fracture with encroachment on the spinal cord may cause morbidity (i.e., paralysis) or death.

Etiology: Fractures to C1 occur as a result of axial loading to the top of the head (e.g., swimming- and diving-related accidents). The degree of injury depends on the magnitude of the axial loading and whether the spine is in flexion, neutral, or an extension position.

Epidemiology: Trauma to the spine occurs more commonly in the cervical region than in any other area of the spine.

Signs and Symptoms: The patient may present with pain or a varying degree of paralysis.

Imaging Characteristics: CT is the modality of choice for the diagnosis of a C1 fracture.

CT
- Noncontrast study with bone window setting shows fracture of the C1 vertebrae.
- May demonstrate other related bony or soft tissue injuries to the upper cervical region.

MRI
- Useful in evaluating the spinal cord and other soft tissue structures of the spine.

Treatment: Most fractures of the C1 vertebrae can be treated with immobilization (e.g., rigid cervical orthosis or a halo vest).

Prognosis: Depends on the degree of injury and other associated injuries.

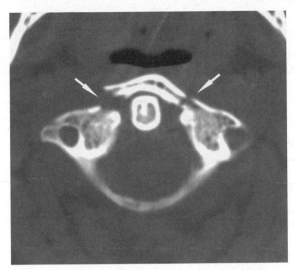

FIGURE 1. **Fracture of C1.** Axial CT of C1 demonstrates fractures of the anterior arch (*arrows*).

Cervical Facet Lock

Description: A dislocation of the zygapophyseal or facet joint of the cervical spine. A facet lock (dislocation or subluxation) occurs when the inferior articulating process (facet) of the superior vertebra is locked in front of the superior articulating process (facet) of the inferior vertebra. A facet lock or facet dislocation may appear either unilateral or bilateral.

Etiology: Motor vehicle accidents (MVA) including motorcycle accidents, falls, and other accidents resulting from recreational activities are the leading causes of injuries to the lower cervical spine. This is usually the result of a flexion/distraction and rotation type of injury.

The position of the head and neck at the time of impact and the direction of the force are key factors in this type of injury.

Epidemiology: Unilateral facet injuries represent 6% to 10% of all cervical spine injuries. Most often occurs at either the C4-5 or C5-6 level.

Signs and Symptoms: Injury to the posterior spinal ligament and spinal instability result in pain, limited rotation motion, and radiculopathy. Bilateral facet dislocations are frequently associated with neurological deficits.

Imaging Characteristics:

CT
- Midline sagittal multiplanar reconstruction (MPR) shows the anterior subluxation of the body of the superior vertebra over the body of the inferior vertebra.
- Parasagittal MPR of the superior and inferior articulating processes are dislocated.
- Axial image shows normal relationship of the inferior and superior facets as the "hamburger on a bun" sign. The locked facet may be seen as the reverse hamburger on a bun sign.

MRI
- Good to show pertinent anatomy of the zygapophyseal joint.
- Disk herniation can be identified.

Treatment: For unilateral facet dislocation, surgical treatment (open reduction) with internal fixation is more successful than closed reduction traction with a halo vest. Bilateral facet dislocation may be more easily reduced with closed traction. They may also redislocate and require internal fixation.

Prognosis: Surgical treatment results in reduced treatment failure, reduced pain, and neurological deterioration as compared to nonsurgical treatment.

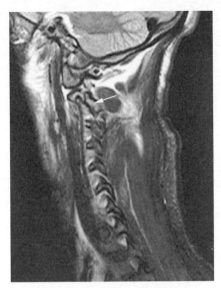

FIGURE 1. Cervical Facet Lock. Sagittal STIR image of a unilateral cervical facet lock with C2 locked on C3 (*arrow*).

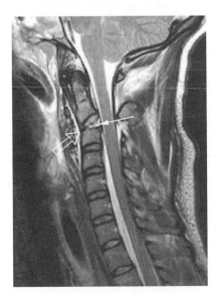

FIGURE 2. Cervical Facet Lock. Midline sagittal T2 -weighted image (same patient as above) showing high signal of C2-C3 disk consistent with an acute injury of the disk (*arrow*). Ligamentous injury is seen anterior to C2-C3 (*open arrow*).

Vertebral Compression Fracture

Description: Compression fractures of the lumbar spine occur as a result of a combination of flexion and axial loading (compression) of the vertebrae.

Etiology: This fracture can occur as a result of trauma, metastatic disease to the spine, or osteoporosis.

Epidemiology: Compression fractures are common in the aging and geriatric patients with osteoporosis.

Signs and Symptoms: Patient presents with back pain and possible neurologic deficit.

Imaging Characteristics: CT is the imaging modality to demonstrate bony anatomy, while MRI is better for showing soft tissue structures and spinal cord.

CT
- Fracture of vertebral body.
- Fractures of the pedicles and lamina.
- Shows displaced fracture fragments that may compromise the spinal canal.
- Thin-section multiplanar images are very useful.

MRI
- Excellent modality to evaluate the status of the spinal canal and spinal cord.
- May show cord hemorrhage.
- May show compromise of the spinal canal and compression of the spinal cord.
- May show associated ligamentous injury or herniated disk.

Treatment: These injuries are usually stable because the bony posterior elements and longitudinal ligaments are intact.

Prognosis: Depends on the extent of the injury and status of the spinal canal and cord.

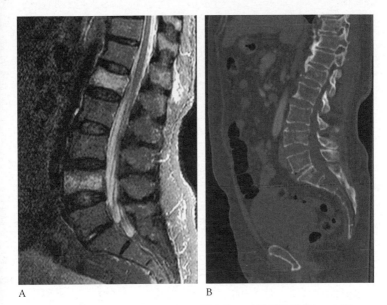

A   B

FIGURE 1. **Compression Fracture L1 and L4.** Sagittal T2W MR (A) and CT sagittal MPR (B) images show compression fractures of L1 and L4, respectively.

Spinal Cord Hematoma

Description: A spinal cord hematoma is a collection of blood in the spinal cord, most commonly due to trauma.

Etiology: Most spinal cord hematomas occur as a result of trauma to the spinal cord, ligamentous structures, and/or bony vertebra. Other associated causes may include an acute herniated disk or hemorrhage from an arteriovenous malformation.

Epidemiology: Trauma to the spinal column occurs at an incidence of approximately 2 to 5 per 100,000 population. Many of these injuries are a result of motor vehicle accidents. Less frequent causes include falls, diving accidents, and sports and recreational injuries. Adolescences and young adults, especially males, are more commonly affected.

Signs and Symptoms: Depending on the level and extent of the injury, the patient may present with motor and sensory dysfunction.

Imaging Characteristics: Plain x-rays of the spine should be done first. CT is good for the evaluation of bony structures, whereas MRI is excellent for the evaluation of soft tissue and spinal cord. Extrinsic changes include disk herniation and ligamentous injury. Intrinsic changes include edema and hemorrhage.

MRI
1. Acute stage (several hours to 3 days)
   - Slightly low signal on T1-weighted images.
   - Marked low signal with high signal on surrounding edema on T2-weighted images.
2. Subacute stage (3 days to 3 weeks)
   - High signal on T1-weighted images.
   - High signal with low signal clot on T2-weighted images.
3. Chronic stage (3 weeks to months)
   - High signal on T1-weighted images.
   - High signal with low-signal rim on T2-weighted images.
   - Gradient echo images appear with low-signal intensity.

Treatment: Presence of a spinal cord hematoma indicates a poor prognosis. Permanent neurologic deficit is most likely.

Prognosis: Depends on the type, level, and extent of the injury.

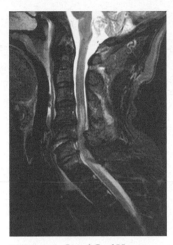

FIGURE 1. Spinal Cord Hematoma.
Sagittal T2W MR image demonstrated
slightly heterogeneous hyperintense
cord signal abnormality consistent with
hematoma and edema.

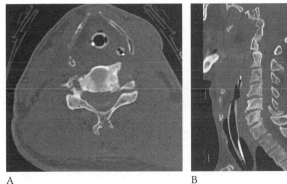

A

B

FIGURE 2. Spinal Cord Hematoma. Axial (A) and sagittal CT (B) images (the same
patient as in Figure 1) through the cervical spine demonstrate a fracture through C5.

Fracture/Dislocation (C6-C7)

Description: Spinal subluxation is the partial dislocation of the spinal vertebrae. Facet dislocations may be either stable (unilateral) or unstable (bilateral) in more severe cases. A subluxation of the spinal vertebrae is associated with either a partial or complete disruption of the posterior longitudinal ligament and the anterior longitudinal ligament. In many cases, this may be associated with a fracture of either facet at the level of the dislocation.

Etiology: Traumatic conditions that result in hyperextension or hyperflexion and rotation of the cervical spine.

Epidemiology: Cervical spine subluxation is associated with hyperextension- and hyperflexion-related traumatic injuries to the cervical column.

Signs and Symptoms: Patient presents with pain and possible neurologic deficit.

Imaging Characteristics: Plain films should be done first for screening.

CT
- Useful in identifying bony injury (fracture), extent of fracture, status of posterior elements and spinal canal.
- Spiral CT (single or multidetector) with thin sections (1 to 3 mm) sagittal and coronal reformatted.

MRI
- Excellent for the evaluation of the spinal cord and other soft tissue injuries.

Treatment: Reduction of the fracture/dislocation.

Prognosis: Depends on the extent of the trauma and status of the spinal cord. The presence of cord hemorrhage is generally considered to be a poor prognosis.

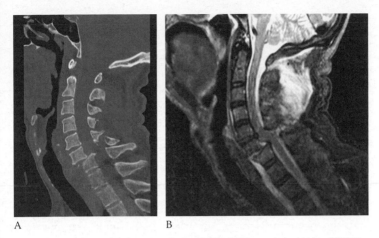

A   B

FIGURE 1. **Fracture/Dislocation.** Sagittal MPR CT bone window (A) and T2W sagittal MR (B) images reveal fracture-dislocation injury of C5-C7 with anterolisthesis of C6 on C7, cord hemorrhage, and ligamentous injury.

Odontoid Fracture

Description: Fractures of the odontoid process or dens have been classi-fied into three types. A Type I fracture, rarely seen, is an avulsion of the tip of the dens. Type II, the most common, consists of a fracture through the base of the dens. Type III fractures extend through the upper body of the C2 vertebrae.

Etiology: Fractures of the dens usually result from extreme flexion of the head.

Epidemiology: Trauma to the spine occurs more commonly in the cervical region than in any other area of the spine.

Signs and Symptoms: Patient may present with pain or a varying degree of neurologic deficit.

Imaging Characteristics: Spiral CT is the modality of choice for the diagnosis of an odontoid fracture.

CT
- Noncontrast study with sagittal and coronal reformatted bone win-dow images shows fracture of the dens.
- May demonstrate other related bony or soft tissue injuries to the upper cervical spine.

MRI
- Useful in evaluating the spinal cord and other soft tissue structures.

Treatment: Depending on the type of fracture, immobilization with a halo vest and possible bony fusion may be successful.

Prognosis: Depends on the type of fracture and status of the spinal cord.

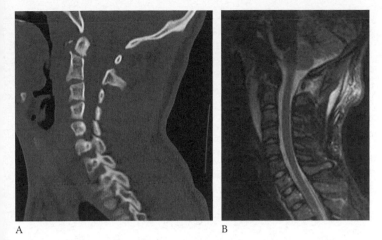

A   B

FIGURE 1. **Fracture of the Odontoid of C2.** CT sagittal MPR (A) bone window and T2W sagittal MR (B) images demonstrate a transverse odontoid (type II) fracture.

SPINE
VASCULAR DISEASE

Spinal Cord Ischemia/Infarction

Description: Ischemia and infarction of the spinal cord is the decrease or absence of blood to the spinal cord.

Etiology: Most result from atherosclerosis, hypertension, thoracoabdominal aortic aneurysm, sickle cell anemia, caisson disease, diabetes, meningitis, and spinal trauma.

Epidemiology: The lower thoracic cord and conus are most commonly involved.

Signs and Symptoms: The patient presents with diminished bowel and bladder function, loss of perineal sensation, and reduced sensory and motor function of the lower extremities.

Imaging Characteristics: MRI is the imaging modality of choice for the diagnosis of spinal cord ischemia or infarction.

MRI
- T1-weighted images may show an enlargement of the spinal cord.
- T2-weighted images show high-signal intensity in the cord.
- FLAIR images are very helpful by suppressing the CSF signal.

Treatment: Treatment is usually symptomatic.

Prognosis: Depends on the extent and severity of the infarct.

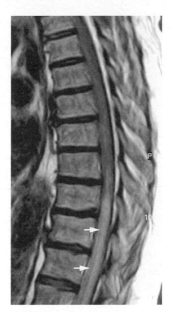

FIGURE 1. **Spinal Cord Ischemia/Infarct.** FLAIR sagittal image of the thoracic spine shows an enlargement with diffuse increased signal intensity (*arrows*) of the distal thoracic spinal cord.

PART IV

Head and Neck

CONGENITAL

Brachial Cleft Cyst

Description: Brachial cleft cysts (BCC) are congenital anomalies and usually arise from the second brachial arch during embryological development. During clinical presentation the cystic mass appears in the anteriolateral portion of the neck around the angle of the mandible.

Etiology: Congenital anomaly.

Epidemiology: Bimodal age distribution. The first occurrence is at birth with the second peak seen in young adults. About 10% are bilateral in location.

Signs and Symptoms: This cystic mass is usually painless.

Imaging Characteristics: Shows well-defined round cystic mass posterolateral to the submandibular gland. There is no contrast enhancement.

CT
◆ Shows cyst as low density.

MRI
◆ T1-weighted (T1W) image is hypointense.
◆ T2-weighted image is hyperintense.

Treatment: Complete surgical resection.

Prognosis: Good.

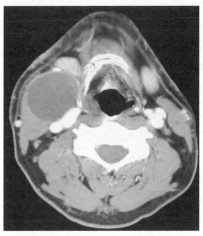

FIGURE 1. Brachial Cleft Cyst. Axial contrast-enhanced computed tomography (CECT) shows a cystic lesion in the right neck of a child located anteromedial to the sternocleidomastoid muscle, posterolateral to the submandibular gland, and lateral to the carotid space. In a child, this is a classic location and appearance for a second type BCC. Other differential considerations would include suppurative lymphadenitis or necrotic lymph node metastases (in an adult).

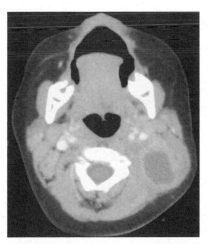

FIGURE 2. Brachial Cleft Cyst. Axial CECT in a child shows a cystic lesion in the left posterior neck with overlying infiltration of the fat representing an inflamed second BCC.

TUMOR

Cavernous Hemangioma (Orbital)

Description: Cavernous hemangiomas of the orbit are the most common benign orbital tumors in adults.

Etiology: These vascular malformations are composed of large dilated endothelium-lined vascular channels covered by a fibrous capsule.

Epidemiology: These slow, progressive tumors usually occur in patients between the second and fourth decades of life and are slightly more common in females. These tumors are usually located intraconal, but extraconal cavernous hemangiomas are possible.

Signs and Symptoms: Patients present with painless proptosis (bulging eyes).

Imaging Characteristics:

CT
- Appear as well-defined, high-density, smooth-margined, homogeneous, rounded, ovoid (egg shaped), or lobulated mass with marked contrast enhancement.

MRI
- T1-weighted images demonstrate an isointense to hypointense well-circumscribed mass.
- The tumor appears hyperintense to fat on T2-weighted images.
- Postcontrast T1-weighted images show marked enhancement.

Treatment: Surgical resection of these encapsulated benign tumors is the recommended treatment of choice.

Prognosis: Surgical resection produces a high cure rate.

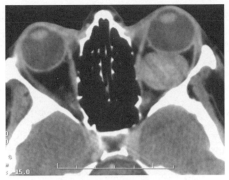

FIGURE 1. Cavernous Hemangioma.
Noncontrast CT showing smoothly marginated, high-density, round, contrast-enhancing intraconal mass of the left orbit displacing the left globe anteriorly.

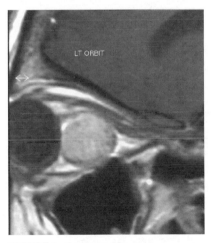

FIGURE 2. Cavernous Hemangioma.
Sagittal T1-weighted postcontrast MR shows round, slightly hyperintense, retrobular mass displacing optic nerve superiorly.

Cholesteatoma (Acquired)

Description: An acquired cholesteatoma consists of an accumulation of squamous epithelium in the middle ear.

Etiology: Varies, depending on the specific type of cholesteatoma.

Epidemiology: Unknown; however, a cholesteatoma is a relatively common reason for ear surgery.

Signs and Symptoms: Most common sign is frequent recurrent painless discharge from the ear. Hearing loss may also be common.

Imaging Characteristics: High-resolution CT (HRCT) is the preferred modality used to evaluate the mass-like lesion in the middle ear which erodes the ossicles and bone.

CT
- Thin section axial and coronal images useful in evaluating temporal bone.
- Useful in planning surgery.
- Can determine extent of cholesteatoma and related structures.
- Acquired temporal bone cholesteatoma characterized by a soft-tissue homogeneous mass with focal bone destruction (erosion).

MRI
- Thin section axial and coronal images useful in evaluating temporal bone.
- Useful in planning surgery.
- Can determine extent of cholesteatoma and related structures.
- Acquired temporal bone cholesteatoma (soft-tissue mass) appears hypointense on T1-weighted images, no enhancement is seen following gadolinium.
- Cholesteatoma is hyperintense on T2-weighted images.

Treatment: Surgical intervention.

Prognosis: Good.

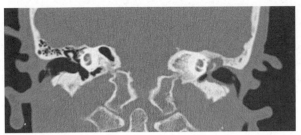

FIGURE 1. Cholesteatoma. Coronal NECT shows soft tissue density in the left middle ear with thickening of the tympanic membrane. The left scutum has a blunted appearance (compared to sharp tip of normal right side). Findings are consistent with a cholesteatoma.

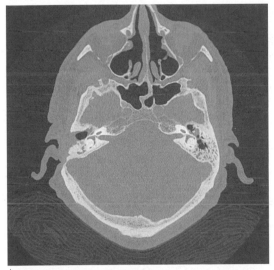

A

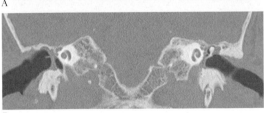

B

FIGURE 2. Cholesteatoma. Axial NECT (A) of the temporal bones shows soft tissue in the left middle ear located lateral to the ossicles in the epitympanum (Prussak space). Mastoidectomy has previously been performed on the right. Coronal CT (B) in same patient shows soft tissue in left middle ear within Prussak space of the epitympanum with blunting of the scutum. Right mastoidectomy is present.

Glomus Tumor (Paraganglioma)

Description: A glomus tumor or paraganglioma is a benign, slow-growing, hypervascular lesion. They are named according to their anatomic location such as *glomus vagale* (most common) when in the carotid space above the carotid bifurcation. Others, such as, *glomus jugulare* are associated with the jugular foramen and *glomus tympanicum* when associated with the middle ear.

Etiology: This is a benign tumor arising from the neural crest paraganglion cells of the extracranial head and neck.

Epidemiology: These lesions may be multiple in 5% of the patients and almost 30% of the patients have a familial history of the disease.

Signs and Symptoms: Depends on the location of the tumor.

Imaging Characteristics:

CT
- Contrast-enhanced study demonstrates an enhancing, well-circumscribed, soft-tissue mass.

MRI
- T1-weighted images show mixed signal intensity mass with multiple signal (flow) voids.
- Paragangliomas produce a high signal on T2-weighted images.
- Postcontrast T1-weighted images of the tumor are hyperintense with signal (flow) voids giving it a salt-and-pepper appearance.

Treatment: May require surgery, radiation therapy, or both.

Prognosis: Good, this is a benign tumor.

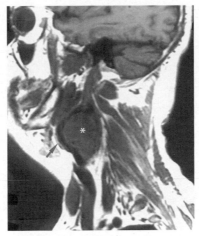

FIGURE 1. Glomus Tumor (Glomus Vagala). T1-weighted left parasagittal image shows an intermediate signal mass (*asterisk*) of the upper neck at the carotid bifurcation. The external carotid artery (*arrow*) is displaced anteriorly.

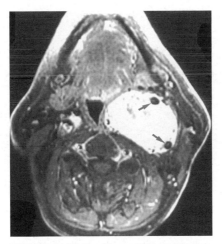

FIGURE 2. Glomus Tumor (Glomus Vagala). Postcontrast T1-weighted axial image shows a large markedly enhancing mass of the upper neck splaying the internal and external (*arrows*) carotids above the common carotid artery bifurcation.

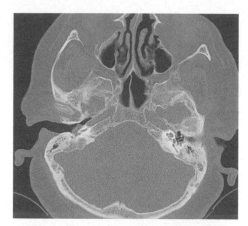

FIGURE 3. Glomus Tumor (Glomus Tympanicum).
Axial CT shows soft tissue in the right middle ear
overlying the cochlear promontory. Permeative bone
loss is seen in the mastoid bone adjacent to the
posterior fossa on the right.

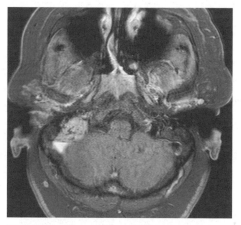

**FIGURE 4. Glomus Tumor (Glomus
Jugulotympanicum).** Axial fat-sat (FS) T1W with
gadolinium shows enhancing mass in right mastoid
region and jugular fossa. Serpentine flow voids
represent vessels.

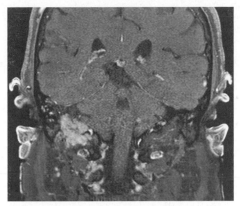

FIGURE 5. **Glomus Tumor (Glomus Jugulotympanicum).** Coronal FS T1W with gadolinium shows enhancing mass extending from right middle ear into jugular fossa representing a glomus jugulotympanicum tumor (paraganglioma).

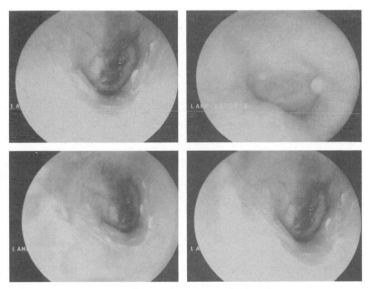

FIGURE 6. **Glomus Tumor (Glomus Tympanicum).** Clinical otoscopic images show a (blue) vascular mass located behind the eardrum. This corresponds to the mass seen on the cochlear promontory (Figure 3). (see Color Insert).

Parotid Gland Tumor (Benign Adenoma)

Description: The salivary glands can be divided into major and minor types. The major salivary glands include the parotid, submandibular, and sublingual glands. The parotid gland is the largest salivary gland and forms the majority of salivary neoplasms. The minor salivary glands are comprised of hundreds of smaller glands distributed throughout the mucosa and aerodigestive tract.

Etiology: Radiation has been suspected as a potential cause of both benign and malignant lesions.

Epidemiology: The average age to acquire a parotid gland tumor is between the fourth and fifth decades of life. Greater than 80% of parotid gland tumors are benign mixed tumors (pleomorphic adenomas). The tendency for malignant tumors increases in the submandibular, sublingual, and the minor salivary glands.

Signs and Symptoms: Benign tumors are usually palpable, discrete, and mobile. Malignant tumors commonly present as a palpable lump or mass. Pain, rapid expansion, poor mobility, and facial nerve weakness are additional symptoms associated with malignancy.

Imaging Characteristics: Mass effect may displace surrounding anatomy.

CT
- Shows round mass with density similar to that of muscle against fatty background of the normal parotid gland.
- Demonstrates mild to moderate contrast enhancement.

MRI
- Lesions are best identified on T1-weighted images amid the bright signal of parotid fat.
- Benign tumors are very bright on T2-weighted images.
- Malignant tumors may have mixed signal intensities on T2-weighted images.

Treatment: Surgical removal for benign tumors. For malignant parotid gland tumors, complete surgical resection with radiation therapy is indicated.

Prognosis: Good; 80% of parotid gland tumors are benign. For those that are malignant, the patient outcome depends on the staging of the cancer and early detection and treatment. The overall 10-year survival rates for stages I, II, and III are approximately 90%, 65%, and 22%, respectively.

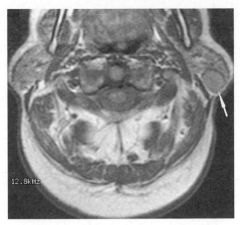

FIGURE 1. Parotid Gland Tumor. T1-weighted axial MRI of the parotid gland demonstrates a well-defined, round, low-signal intensity mass (*arrow*) in the posterior aspect of the superficial lobe of the left parotid gland.

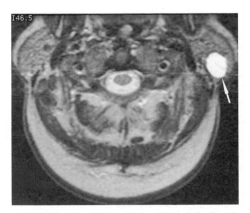

FIGURE 2. Parotid Gland Mass. T2-weighted axial MRI of the parotid gland demonstrates a well-defined high-signal intensity mass (*arrow*) of the posterior aspect of the superficial lobe of the left parotid gland consistent with a pleomorphic adenoma.

Thyroid Goiter

Description: Enlargement of the thyroid gland causing a swelling in the anterior portion of the neck. This type of goiter may also be referred to as a nontoxic goiter which is not related to an over production of thyroid hormone or malignancy.

Etiology: In the United States, this is more commonly from an increase in thyroid-stimulating hormone (TSH) due to a defect in normal hormone synthesis within the thyroid gland.

Epidemiology: May occur in 1% to 10% of the population.

Signs and Symptoms: Visible swelling in the anterior base of the neck, coughing, difficulty in swallowing (dysphagia), and difficulty in breathing (dyspnea). Nontoxic goiters are slow growing.

Imaging Characteristics:

CT
- Normal thyroid gland appears just below the level of the cricoid cartilage.
- Normal thyroid gland appears as two wedge-shaped structures just lateral to the trachea with homogeneous attenuation on noncontrast examination.
- Good to evaluate anatomy of the neck.
- Good to show compression or deviation of the trachea.
- Good to show intrathoracic extension of the goiter.

MRI
- Normal thyroid gland appears with intermediate signal on T1-weighted images.
- Normal thyroid gland appears with higher signal on T2-weighted images.
- Good to evaluate anatomy of the neck.
- Good to show compression or deviation of the trachea.
- Good to show intrathoracic extension of the goiter.

Treatment: Thyroid hormone suppressive therapy; thyroxine (T4) therapy may reduce the size of the goiter. Surgical removal or decompression results in quick relief of obstructive symptoms.

Prognosis: Good.

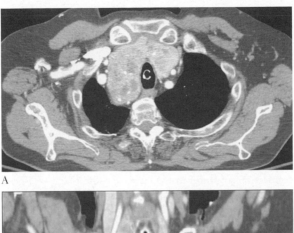

A

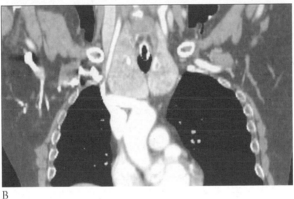

B

FIGURE 1. **Thyroid Goiter.** Axial (A) and coronal (B) CECTs show an enlarged heterogeneously enhancing thyroid gland with multiple low-attenuation cysts and calcifications, respectively.

INFECTION

Peritonsillar Abscess

Description: Peritonsillar abscess (PTA) is an accumulation of pus in the tonsillar bed with medial displacement of the tonsil.

Etiology: May be caused by a viral or bacterial infection.

Epidemiology: Peritonsillar abscesses make up approximately 50% of head and neck infections in children. PTAs most commonly occur between the ages of 20 and 40 years. Males and females are equally affected.

Signs and Symptoms: Common findings include progressively worsening sore throat (often localized to one side), pain (suggests the location of the abscess), painful and difficult swallowing, fever, dysphagia, and earache.

Imaging Characteristics:

CT
- Helpful in determining the degree of airway compromise.
- Determine the location of the abscess.
- Identify the proximity of the internal carotid artery and internal jugular vein in preparation for needle aspiration on deep abscesses.
- PTAs appear diffuse and as ill-defined thickening in the tonsillar region.
- NECT inflammatory process appears hypodense to isodense.
- Contrast-enhanced CT shows loss of fat planes and edema in surrounding area.
- Contrast-enhanced CT shows abscess as a cystic/mutilocular hypodense collection with rim enhancement, with or without the presence of gas at the center.

MRI
- T1-weighted images appear hypointense to isointense to surrounding muscles.
- Hyperintense on T2-weighted images.
- Gadolinium-based T1-weighted images show enhancing rim of abscess.

Treatment: The gold standard of treatment is to perform a peritonsillar aspiration and antibiotic therapy. In advance cases a tonsillectomy may be required.

Prognosis: Good; however, there is a risk of 10% to 30% of developing a secondary PTA.

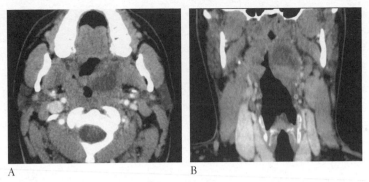

A   B

FIGURE 1. Peritonsillar Abscess. Axial (A) and coronal (B) CECTs show low attenuation with minimal rim enhancement in left tonsillar region representing phlegmon or early abscess of the faucial tonsil.

Submandibular Salivary Gland Abscess

Description: Submandibular salivary gland abscesses are mucus-filled retention cysts derived from obstructed or traumatized salivary ducts.

Etiology: May be caused by a stone in the submandibular duct, or in the gland itself. Inflammation of the submandibular lymph nodes may arise secondary to a dental abscess, or an infective lesion of the tongue, floor of the mouth, mandible, cheek, or neighboring skin.

Epidemiology: Unknown.

Signs and Symptoms: Abscesses are associated with skin thickening, edema of the fat, and gas in over 50% of cases. They are also associated with pain and tenderness in the area of the affected gland.

Imaging Characteristics:

CT
- Low-density cystic mass.
- May show variable contrast enhancement.

MRI
- Hypointense on T1-weighted images.
- Hyperintense on T2-weighted images.

Treatment: Submandibular swelling may be treated with antibiotics. Surgical intervention may be required in select cases.

Prognosis: Good with early diagnosis and treatment.

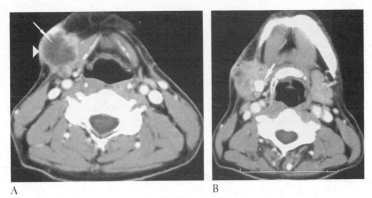

A

B

FIGURE 1. **Abscess of the Submandibular Salivary Gland.** In (A), postcontrast CT shows enlarged right submandibular gland with central low density (*small arrow*) and irregular peripheral contrast enhancement (*arrowhead*). Postcontrast axial CT (B) image demonstrates a calcified stone (*arrow*) in the right submandibular gland. These findings are consistent with an abscess of the right submandibular gland secondary to an obstruction from a stone (calculus).

SINUS

Mucocele

Description: Mucoceles arise as a complication associated with sinusitis. They are the most common expansive lesions involving the paranasal sinuses.

Etiology: Mucoceles tend to occur as a consequence of a long-standing obstruction of the paranasal sinuses.

Epidemiology: Mucoceles most commonly affect the frontal sinus. Maxillary and ethmoid sinuses combined comprise approximately a third of all mucoceles. The sphenoid sinus is rarely involved.

Signs and Symptoms: Since mucoceles are noninfected lesions, they typically present clinically with symptoms associated with mass effect.

Imaging Characteristics:

CT
- Complete opacification and expansion of the sinus with thinned walls.
- There may be bony erosion of the sinus wall.

MRI
- Most appear low signal intensity on T1-weighted images and high signal intensity on T2-weighted images.
- Some may appear dilated but aerated (inspissated) and are hypointense on both T1- and T2-weighted images.

Treatment: Surgical drainage of the sinus cavity.

Prognosis: Good with early diagnosis and treatment.

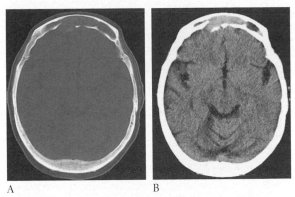

FIGURE 1. Mucocele. Axial NECTs in bone (A) and brain (B) windows show a mass filling the frontal sinus with bony destruction of the posterior wall of the frontal sinus with intracranial extension.

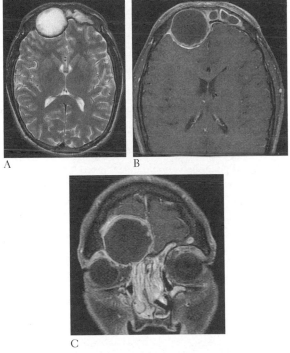

FIGURE 2. Mucocele. T2 axial image (A) shows hyperintense mass that has caused smooth bony remodeling of the right frontal sinus. There is a hypointense rim surrounding the trapped fluid representing the thin bony wall and capsule. Axial (B) and coronal (C) FS T1W images with gadolinium show thin enhancement of the wall of the mucocele with no central enhancement. Patient subsequently underwent neurosurgical evacuation of the mucocele.

Sinusitis

Description: Sinusitis is an acute or chronic inflammation of the paranasal sinuses.

Etiology: Bacterial, viral, or fungal infections may cause sinusitis.

Epidemiology: All ages can be affected. Males and females are equally affected.

Signs and Symptoms: Nasal congestion, a feel of pressure building around the orbital area and associated headache, malaise, and fever are common indicators of sinusitis. Patients may also experience sore throat or an occasional cough.

Imaging Characteristics: Coronal CT is the best imaging plane for the evaluation of sinus diseases.

CT

- Examination of the sinuses reveals mucosal thickening, opacification, or air-fluid levels in one or more of the paranasal sinuses.
- CT also shows obliteration of osteomental complex (common drainage area for frontal anterior ethmoid and maxillary sinuses).

Treatment: Steam inhalation may aid the patient in providing comfort and encourage drainage. Antibiotics, analgesics, and antihistamines may also be used to treat sinusitis. Preventative measures include allergy testing, avoid cigarette smoking, and avoid extreme changes in temperature.

Prognosis: A good prognosis should be expected.

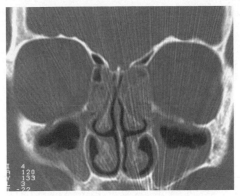

FIGURE 1. Sinusitis. Coronal CT of the sinuses shows moderate thickening of the bilateral maxillary sinuses and marked opacification of the bilateral ethmoid sinuses. There is obliteration of the bilateral osteomental complex.

TRAUMA

Intraocular Foreign Body

Description: An intraocular foreign body is one of several injuries that may result from ocular trauma. An intraocular foreign body occurs as a result of an object penetrating and remaining in the orbit.

Ocular trauma may result from any of the following: (1) globe disruption, (2) lens dislocation, (3) intraocular foreign body, or (4) hemorrhage. In the case of an intraocular foreign body, an object has penetrated the orbit.

Etiology: Injuries may occur at home, in the workplace, during recreation, or as auto accidents. Many injuries are occupationally related, such as metal workers and construction workers. In some cases, injuries may result from BB guns or other small projectile objects.

Epidemiology: Males are more commonly affected than females. All ages can be affected; however, the median age is in the second and third decades of life.

Signs and Symptoms: The patient usually states "something has hit them in the eye." Pain and discomfort are the initial symptoms.

Imaging Characteristics:

CT
- Shows opaque foreign bodies in the orbit.
- Shows bony fractures in the orbital area.
- Shows hemorrhage in the orbital area.

MRI
- The presence of an intraocular metallic foreign body is a contraindication to performing an MRI due to the possibility of an ocular injury occurring from movement of a ferromagnetic substance.

Treatment: Surgery is usually required.

Prognosis: Good, if the foreign body is outside the globe.

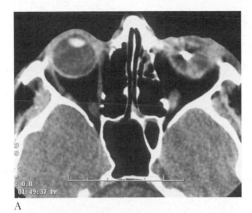

A

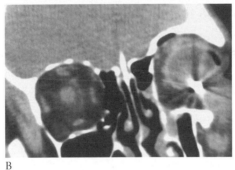

B

FIGURE 1. **Intraocular Foreign Body.** Axial (A) and coronal (B) noncontrast CTs of the orbits demonstrate a small metallic foreign body within the inferior aspect of the left globe. There is no evidence of hemorrhage. Note: There are metallic artifacts from the foreign body.

Tripod Fracture

Description: The tripod fracture is the most common facial fracture. It is comprised of three fractures involving the zygomatic arch, orbital floor or rim, and the maxillary process.

Etiology: This injury results from a blunt force blow to the area of the zygoma.

Epidemiology: It may happen to anyone who experiences a blunt force blow to the area of the zygoma.

Signs and Symptoms: Pain and swelling in the "cheek" area of the face, bruising, and facial disfigurement.

Imaging Characteristics:

CT

- CT is the preferred modality.
- Axial and coronal images are needed for the evaluation of the full extent of the injury.
- Shows fractures of the zygomatic arch, posterolateral wall of the maxillary sinus, and the orbital floor and rim.
- Opacification of maxillary sinus, secondary to blood.

Treatment: Surgery is usually required.

Prognosis: Depends on the extent of the injury and other associated injuries (i.e., brain hemorrhage).

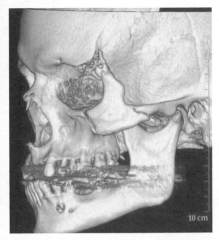

FIGURE 1. Tripod Fracture. CT 3D reformatted shows fracture of the zygomatic arch, zygomaticofrontal suture, and zygomaticomaxillary suture, the three components of a tripod or zygomaticomaxillary (ZMC) fracture complex.

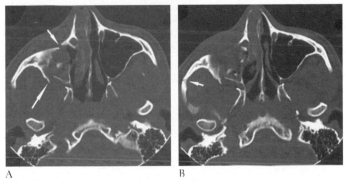

A   B

FIGURE 2. Tripod Fracture. Axial CT of facial bones (A) demonstrates fractures of the anterior (*small arrow*) and posterolateral (*large arrow*) walls of the right maxillary sinus. In (B) there is also a *fracture* of the right zygomatic arch (*arrow*).

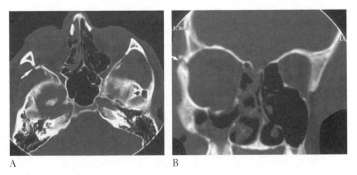

A   B

FIGURE 3. Tripod Fracture. Axial (A) and coronal CTs (B) of the facial bones show a fracture of the lateral wall of the right orbit (*arrow*) and diastasis (separation) of the right frontozygomatic suture, respectively.

PART V

Chest and Mediastinum

CARDIAC

Aberrant Right Subclavian Artery

Description: An aberrant right subclavian artery, also known as arteria lusoria, is an anomaly of the right subclavian artery. It arises directly from the aortic arch instead of originating from the brachiocephalic artery. More specifically, it arises as the fourth branch after the left subclavian artery. The branches then would be identified in order as the right common carotid artery, the left common carotid artery, the left subclavian artery, and the right subclavian artery. This is the most common aortic arch anomaly.

Note: The historical origin of the term arteria lusoria, also known as dysphagia lusoria, dates back to the 1700s. Its discovery during autopsy was accidental and called a "freak of nature," thus the term "lusoria." To read more about the initial discovery look for "David Bayford. His Syndrome and Sign of Dysphagia Lusoria" in the *Annals of the Royal College of Surgeons of England* (1979), volume 61.

Etiology: Occurs early during embryologic development.

Epidemiology: The most common anomaly of the branching of the aortic arch is a left aortic arch with an aberrant right subclavian artery branching off the aortic arch. Though this is the most common aortic arch anomaly, it is a rare anomaly with an estimated incidence of 0.5% to 2% of the general population.

Signs and Symptoms: May be asymptomatic, however individuals may experience dysphagia lusoria, retrosternal pain, chronic cough, difficulty in swallowing, and weight loss.

Image Characteristics: Approximately 80% course posterior to the esophagus, while 15% pass between the esophagus and trachea. The remaining 5% pass anterior to the trachea.

CT and MRI
- Shows the aberrant subclavian artery branching from the aortic arch.
- Can be useful in determining extrinsic airway compression.
- A Kommerell diverticulum may be seen. This is a bulbous enlargement of the proximal subclavian artery at its origin from the aortic arch, posterior to the esophagus.

Treatment: There are a variety of surgical procedures which may be helpful.

Prognosis: Good.

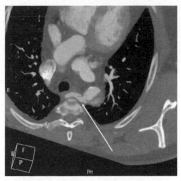

FIGURE 1. Aberrant Right Subclavian Artery. Axial contrast-enhanced CT shows aberrant right subclavian artery moving toward the right arm crossing the midline of the body (*arrow*).

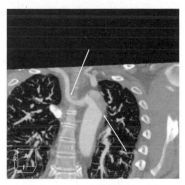

FIGURE 2. Aberrant Right Subclavian Artery. Coronal contrast-enhanced CT shows aberrant right subclavian artery (*top arrow*). Type B aortic dissection involving the descending thoracic aorta extending up to the left subclavian artery is also seen (*bottom arrow*).

Aortic Regurgitation

Description: Aortic regurgitation (AR) is the leakage of or backward flow of blood from the aorta into the left ventricle (LV) through the aortic valve.

Etiology: The two most common causes of acute AR are infective endocarditis and prosthetic valve dysfunction. Post transcatheter aortic valve replacement (TAVR) AR and complications associated with left ventricle assist device (LVAD) implantation have emerged as potential causes of developing aortic regurgitation. Other causes include valvular disease, congenital bicuspid aortic valve, and Marfan syndrome.

Worldwide, rheumatic fever is the most common cause of AR.

Epidemiology: The incidence of AR increases with age, typically peaking in the fourth to sixth decades of life. It occurs more common in males than females.

Signs and Symptoms: Shortness of breath, chest pain, and palpitations may be experienced.

Imaging Characteristics:

CT
- Cardiac CT good for preoperative planning for TAVR, also known as transcatheter aortic valve implantation (TAVI).
- Multiplanar reconstruction (MPR) good to assess cardiac anatomy.
- Use of iterative reconstruction (IR) technology can be used to reduce radiation dose.

MRI
- Cardiac MR (CMR) can be used to evaluate AR severity and LV volumes and function.
- CMR quantitative flow measurement can calculate the regurgitation ejection fraction (EF) to assess AR.
- Signal void known as "jet" emanating from the valve is helpful in diagnosing stenosis and regurgitation.

Treatment: Surgical intervention is usually indicated; however, the patient may be treated medically with medication.

Prognosis: Depends on the function of the LV and overall health of the patient.

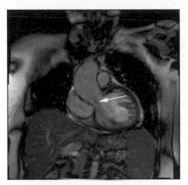

FIGURE 1. Aortic Regurgitation.
Coronal oblique view shows moderate jet
(dark, signal void) emanating from the
aortic value into the left ventricle (*arrow*).
There is also dilatation of the ascending
aorta.

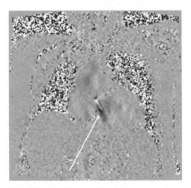

FIGURE 2. Aortic Regurgitation.
Velocity encoded coronal image shows
aortic regurgitation jet into the left
ventricle (*arrow*).

Atrial Myxoma

Description: Benign and malignant tumors of the heart are rare. A myxoma is the most common benign tumor of the heart. Most myxomas (75%) are located in the left atrium (LA). Myxomas may also be found in the right atrium (RA) (18%), right ventricle (RV) (4%), and in the left ventricle (LV) (3%).

Etiology: Cardiac myxoma is a primary tumor that develops mostly in the LA. A low percentage of myxomas may be familial (inherited) and cause symptoms at a younger age.

Epidemiology: Most myxomas are found in patients between 30 and 60 years of age, however, they may be found in people of all ages. Children have a higher incidence of ventricle myxomas than adults. Women are more affected than males. About 5% to 10% of cardiac myxoma patients show familial pattern of tumor development.

Signs and Symptoms: Dyspnea on exertion, paroxysmal nocturnal dyspnea (difficulty breathing while asleep), orthopnea (ability to breathe easily only in the upright position), chest pain or tightness, dizziness, fainting, or palpitations.

Imaging Characteristics: There is a predilection for pedunculated attachment to the interatrial septum, with the majority arising from an area immediately adjacent to the fossa ovalis. Tumor may prolapse through the mitral valve to obstruct outflow of blood.

CT
- Cardiac CT can accurately differentiate and assess cardiac tumors.

MRI
- Cardiac MR can accurately differentiate and assess cardiac tumors.
- Hypointense to myocardium on T1-weighted images.
- Hyperintense on T2-weighted images.
- Steady-state free precession (SSFP) images will show myxoma hyperintense to myocardium, but hypointense to blood pool.
- Heterogeneous enhancement following gadolinium.

Treatment: Surgery is required to remove the entire tumor to reduce the chance of recurrence.

Prognosis: A myxoma is benign. Left untreated, it can lead to embolism or block blood flow as it continues to grow.

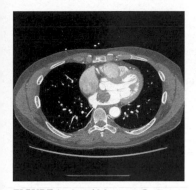

FIGURE 1. Atrial Myxoma. Contrast-enhanced axial CT shows a round filling defect/mass in the left atrium consistent with a myxoma (*arrow*).

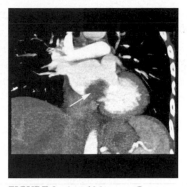

FIGURE 2. Atrial Myxoma. Contrast-enhanced coronal MPR CT shows a round filling defect/mass in the left atrium consistent with a myxoma (*arrow*).

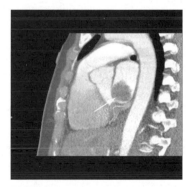

FIGURE 3. Atrial Myxoma. Contrast-enhanced sagittal MPR CT shows a round filling defect/mass in the left atrium consistent with a myxoma (*arrow*).

Coronary Artery Disease

Description: Coronary artery disease (CAD) occurs when atherosclerotic plaque (fatty deposits) builds up in the lumen of the coronary arteries. This disease results in a reduced or absent blood flow to the heart.

Etiology: Atherosclerotic buildup of fatty deposits (plaques) within the lumen of the coronary arteries. This results in a narrowing of the vessel and reduced blood flow.

Epidemiology: This is the most common type of heart disease affecting men and women.

Signs and Symptoms: Most common symptom is angina. Other symptoms include shortness of breath, heart palpitations, tachycardia, weakness or dizziness, nausea, and sweating.

Imaging Characteristics:

CT
- CT angiography (CTA) with IV contrast good to evaluate coronary artery to see if the vessel is occluded.
- Calcium scoring without IV contrast shows calcified plaques.

MRI
- Cardiovascular magnetic resonance (CMR) good to evaluate coronary artery to see if the vessel is occluded.

Treatment: Interventional procedures (e.g., balloon angioplasty, atherectomy, laser treatment, stent placement) may be used. Coronary bypass surgery may be used in select cases.

Prognosis: Depends on the patient's recovery. Change in lifestyle increases better recovery.

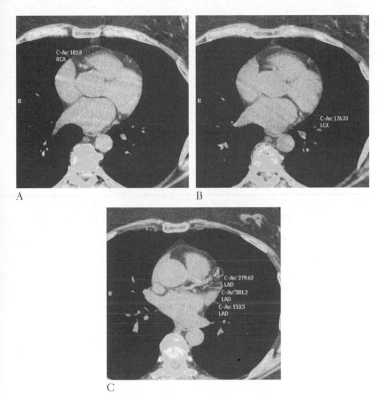

FIGURE 1. Coronary Artery Disease. Nonenhanced CT (NECT) shows computer-aided detection and calculation of coronary artery calcification in the right coronary artery (A), left circumflex artery (B), and left anterior descending coronary artery (C).

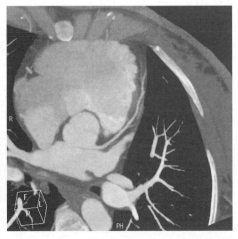

FIGURE 2. Coronary Artery Disease. Maximum intensity projection CT coronary angiogram showing near-complete occlusion of the right coronary artery.

Pericardial Effusion

Description: This condition is defined as a collection of fluid in the pericardial sac.

Etiology: Causative factors may include infections, inflammation, immunologic, traumatic, uremic, neoplastic, hypothyroidism, chylopericarditis, and congestive heart failure.

Epidemiology: Majority of cases are related to known or suspected underlying processes which result from secondary diseases.

Signs and Symptoms: Chest pain, dyspnea, and lightheadedness.

Imaging Characteristics: Ultrasound is the imaging modality of choice.

CT
- Good to differentiate between fluid and blood (hemopericardium).
- Can detect pericardial calcifications.
- Normal pericardial thickness is 3 mm.
- Pericardial thickness greater than 4 mm is suggestive of pericardial thickening.
- Pericarditis may be hyperdense on IV contrast examination.

MRI
- Normal pericardial thickness is 3 mm.
- Pericardial thickness greater than 4 mm is suggestive of pericardial thickening.
- CMR can assess ventricular filling patterns.

Treatment: Many patients require pericardiocentesis to treat or prevent cardiac tamponade while other patients will need surgical intervention.

Prognosis: This is a serious condition and patients should be hospitalized until the treatment is accomplished or symptoms improve.

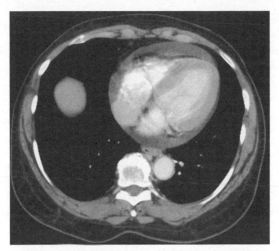

FIGURE 1. **Pericardial Effusion.** Contrast-enhanced CT (CECT) shows increased fluid density around the heart consistent with a pericardial effusion.

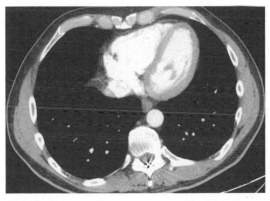

FIGURE 2. **Pericardial Effusion.** Normal for comparison.

Situs Inversus

Description: Situs inversus or dextrocardia (cardiac apex pointing to the right) occurs when the morphologic right atrium is located on the left side of the patient, and the morphologic left atrium is located on the right side of the patient. Situs inversus totalis is a complete right-to-left reversal (transposition) of the thoracic and abdominal organs.

Etiology: Congenital.

Epidemiology: Occurs in about 0.1% of the population. Situs inversus with dextrocardia is more common and 3% to 5% have congenital heart disease. Most of these patients will have a right-sided aortic arch. Situs inversus with levocardia is rare and is usually associated with congenital heart disease.

Signs and Symptoms: Usually asymptomatic. However, some patients, approximately 25%, may have an underlying condition called primary ciliary dyskinesia (PCD), also known as Kartagener syndrome. Kartagener syndrome is characterized as situs inversus, bronchiectasis, and chronic sinus infections.

Imaging Characteristics:

CT
- Preferred modality to diagnose situs inversus with dextrocardia.
- Shows good anatomic detail of organ position and great vessel branching.

MRI
- Useful for difficult cases and with associated cardiac anomalies.

Treatment: No treatment.

Prognosis: Good.

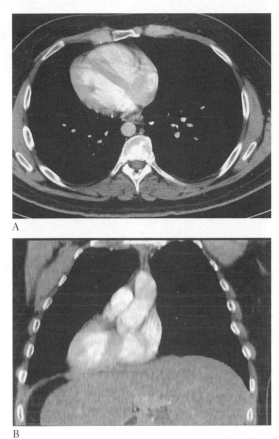

A

B

FIGURE 1. **Situs Inversus.** CT axial (A) and coronal multiplanar reconstruction (MPR) (B) show the heart apex on the right.

Superior Vena Cava Syndrome

Description: This syndrome is the result of an obstruction of blood flow through the superior vena cava (SVC).

Etiology: May be caused from radiation, cannulation (e.g., central venous catheters), tumor bulk, adenopathy, or fibrosing mediastinitis.

Epidemiology: Majority of cases involve malignant mediastinal tumors.

Signs and Symptoms: Dyspnea is the most common symptom. Other symptoms include cough, head and neck fullness, and headache.

Imaging Characteristics:

CT
- Initial test of choice to determine the cause of an obstruction.
- Obstruction of SVC with multiple collateral veins.
- SVC thrombosis.
- Mediastinal tumor obstructing the SVC.

MRI
- Good alternative for patients who may be allergic to iodinated contrast or have renal failure.

Treatment: Depends on the cause. Initial treatment focus is to relieve symptoms. Radiation therapy and chemotherapy may be used to treat tumors. Thrombolytics may be used to treat a thrombus. Surgery may be useful in select cases.

Prognosis: Primarily depends on the cause and course of treatment.

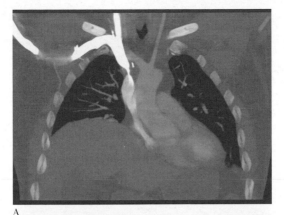

A

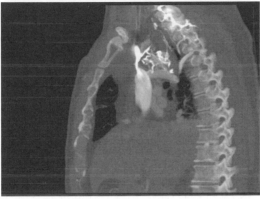

B

FIGURE 1. **Superior Vena Cava Syndrome.** CECT coronal (A) and MPR CECT sagittal (B) images show significant narrowing of the superior vena cava with development of multiple collaterals.

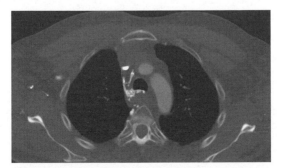

FIGURE 2. **Superior Vena Cava Syndrome.** Axial CECT shows significant narrowing of the superior vena cava with development of multiple collaterals.

INFECTION

Histoplasmosis

Description: A fungal infection affecting the pulmonary system.

Etiology: *Histoplasma capsulatum* (*H. capsulatum*) is the fungal organism which causes histoplasmosis. The organism enters the body through the lungs.

Epidemiology: It is endemic in the Ohio, Missouri, and Mississippi river valley areas. This is the most common endemic fungal infection seen in humans.

Signs and Symptoms: Majority of patients are asymptomatic. For cases where symptoms occur, they may include fever, shortness of breath, pneumonia, muscle aches, headaches, chills, and loss of appetite.

Imaging Characteristics:

CT
- Good to see calcified granulomas in the lung.
- Good to see hilar and mediastinal lymphadenopathy.
- Useful in evaluating patients with mediastinal fibrosis as an ill-defined soft-tissue mass surrounding the trachea.
- Noncalcified granuloma may be difficult to differentiate from neoplastic lesion.

Treatment: Antifungal medication may be used.

Prognosis: Depends on the severity of the disease. As severity of the disease increases, so does the chance that lifelong problems will increase.

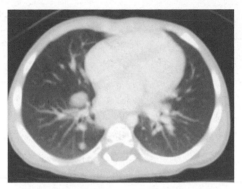

FIGURE 1. **Histoplasmosis.** Axial CECT shows two well-ground glass nodules in the right mid lung in a patient with histoplasmosis.

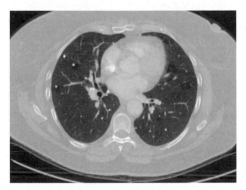

FIGURE 2. **Histoplasmosis.** Axial CT shows multiple well-defined subcentimeter calcified nodules in the lungs and mediastinum as a result of prior histoplasmosis infection.

LUNGS

Adult Respiratory Distress Syndrome

Description: Adult respiratory distress syndrome (ARDS) is characterized by diffuse lung disease. ARDS is described as an acute condition characterized by bilateral pulmonary infiltrates and severe hypoxemia without any evidence of cardiogenic pulmonary edema.

Etiology: Breathing vomit (aspiration pneumonia) into the lungs, pneumonia, septic shock, and trauma may be associated with diffuse alveolar damage.

Epidemiology: It is estimated that about 190,000 cases exist annually in the United States with about 74,500 deaths. Male and females are equally affected. ARDS may occur at any age; however, the incidence rate tends to increase with age.

Signs and Symptoms: Labored, rapid breathing, low blood pressure, and shortness of breath. Hypoxemia may result in organ (liver and kidney) failure.

Imaging Characteristics:

CT
- Diffuse bilateral alveolar lung infiltrate mimicking pulmonary edema or bilateral pneumonia.
- Good in detecting pulmonary interstitial emphysema, pneumothorax and pneumomediastinum, pleural effusions, cavitation, and mediastinal lymphadenopathy.

Treatment: Treatment is focused on underlying conditions, supportive care, and appropriate ventilator and fluid management.

Prognosis: The prognosis has improved in the past several years with 60% to 70% survival. Mortality rate increases in patients older than 65 years and especially those with an underlying condition such as sepsis.

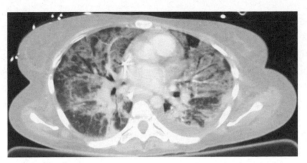

FIGURE 1. CECT shows extensive ground glass opacification of the lungs, with intense parenchymal opacification and air bronchograms. A left pleural effusion is also present.

Asbestosis

Description: A respiratory disease which results from the inhalation (pneumoconiosis) of asbestos fibers. There are two major types of asbestos fibers: (1) amphiboles (crocidolite—stiff and straight) and (2) serpentines (chrysolite—curly and flexible). Exposure to asbestosis also associated with lung cancer and mesothelioma.

Etiology: Inhalation of asbestos.

Epidemiology: Individuals who have worked (occupational exposure) in an asbestos-related occupation are at greatest risk.

Signs and Symptoms: Shortness of breath is usually the first sign. Respiratory infections and coughing up blood occur as the disease progresses.

Imaging Characteristics:

CT
- High-resolution CT (HRCT) more sensitive and specific than conventional radiographs in seeing pleural plaques, pleural thickening, and pleural calcifications.
- HRCT shows interlobular and intralobular septal thickening, ground-glass opacities, and honeycomb pattern.
- Fibrosis typically patchy and similar to usual interstitial pneumonia (UIP).

Treatment: No effective treatment is currently available. For idiopathic pulmonary fibrosis (IPF), home oxygen and prevention of pulmonary infections are recommended.

Prognosis: Poor.

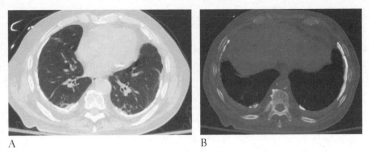

A   B

FIGURE 1. Lung (A) and bone (B) window NECTs of the chest show bilateral calcified pleural plaques and pleural thickening.

Bronchogenic Carcinoma

Description: Lung cancer is one of the various primary malignant neoplasms that may appear in the lung. Lung cancer is the leading cause of death from cancer in both men and women.

Etiology: The exact cause of lung cancer is unknown; however, inhalation of carcinogens is known to be a predisposing cause. Cigarette smoking is by far the most important risk factor for the development of carcinoma of the lung.

Epidemiology: Lung cancer is rarely found in individuals younger than the age of 40. The incidence rate rises rapidly after the age of 50, with 60 years being the average age of occurrence. The majority of cases appear between 50 and 75 years of age. The male-to-female occurrence ratio is 2:1.

Signs and Symptoms: Patients may present with any combination of the following: cough; hemoptysis; dyspnea; pneumonia; chest, shoulder, or arm pain; weight loss; bone pain; hoarseness; headaches; seizures; or swelling of face or neck.

Imaging Characteristics: Chest x-ray is usually done first, although there is some debate regarding spiral CT for screening of lung cancer.

CT
- Appears as a mass with irregular speculated margins.
- There may be central necrosis with large tumors.
- CT is good for staging of lung cancer (i.e., metastatic mediastinal lymph nodes, liver, and adrenal metastasis).

Treatment: Surgery, radiation therapy, and chemotherapy may be used depending on the stage and type of cancer.

Prognosis: Depending on the stage of the cancer, the 5-year survival rate varies from just greater than 50% for patients with stage I to approximately 15% for those with stage III disease.

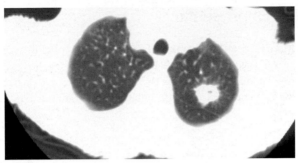

FIGURE 1. Carcinoma of the Lung. CT of the chest with lung windows demonstrates a round mass with irregular speculated margins in the left upper lobe.

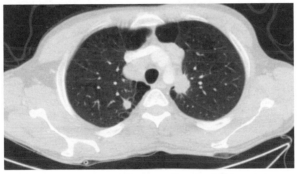

FIGURE 2. Bronchogenic Carcinoma. CT of the chest with lung windows shows bilateral round pulmonary nodules with irregular speculated margins.

Bullous Emphysema

Description: Emphysema is one of the many chronic obstructive pulmonary diseases affecting the lungs. Emphysema involves the destruction of the alveolar wall. This reduces the surface area for gas exchange and allows the collection of free air on inhalation to accumulate in the lung tissue.

Etiology: Cigarette smoking is the most common cause associated with the development of this disease. In a rare form of emphysema, a congenital deficiency in the production of the protein alpha-antitrypsin is associated with the development of emphysema in young adults.

Epidemiology: It is estimated that over 60,000 deaths per year are related to emphysema. Emphysema usually occurs after the fourth decade of life and is more commonly seen in males.

Signs and Symptoms: Patients will typically present with dyspnea, chronic cough, weight loss, malaise, barrel chest, pursed lip breathing, minimal wheezing, and the use of accessory muscles to assist respiration.

Imaging Characteristics:

CT
- Hyperinflation of the lungs.
- Lucent, hypodense (dark) areas of the lung surrounded by normal lung parenchyma. These hypodense sharply demarcated areas measuring 1 cm or greater in diameter are commonly referred to as blebs or bullae and represent the collection of "free air" trapped within the lung during the breathing (inhalation) process and unable to be exhaled.

Treatment: Smoking cessation, administration of oxygen, and eating a well-balanced diet are common methods of treatment. Lung reduction surgery may be indicated in select cases.

Prognosis: Depends on the extent of the disease; however, an improved prognosis is expected if the patient quits smoking, eats a balanced diet, and uses supplemental oxygen.

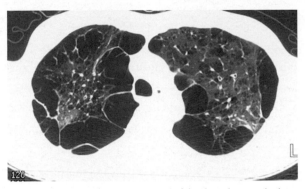

FIGURE 1. Bullous Emphysema. CT of the chest shows multiple bullae of the bilateral upper lobes in the subpleural location.

Mesothelioma

Description: The only major primary malignancy of the mesothelium (membrane covering an internal organ, e.g., lung pleura) of the pleural space.

Etiology: History of inhaling asbestos particles.

Epidemiology: About 70% to 80% of all cases involve a history of asbestos exposure.

Signs and Symptoms: Persistent chest pain and shortness of breath are most common.

Imaging Characteristics:

CT
- Helpful in staging and follow-up.
- Contrast-enhanced CT used to assess tumor response to chemotherapy.
- Difficult to stage in early phase of the disease.
- Calcified pleural plaques indicate prior asbestosis exposure.

MRI
- Difficult to stage in early phase of the disease.

Treatment: Surgery, radiation therapy, chemotherapy, or a combination is used depending on factors such as the location and stage of the cancer.

Prognosis: Poor.

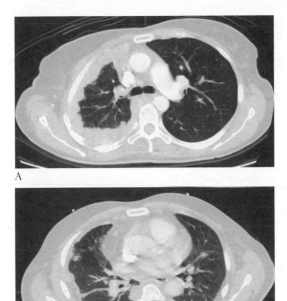

A

B

FIGURE 1. Mesothelioma. Axial CT images of the chest show lobulated plural thickening encasing the right lung and extending along the major fissure.

Pleural Effusion

Description: An abnormal collection of fluid in the pleural space.

Etiology: Results from a variety of diseases such as congestive heart failure (CHF), bacterial infection, malignancy (e.g., lung cancer), and pulmonary embolus.

Epidemiology: Approximately 1.5 million cases are estimated to occur annually in the United States.

Signs and Symptoms: Most common symptoms include dyspnea, cough, and chest pain. Other symptoms may be seen depending on the underlying disease process.

Imaging Characteristics:

CT
- Best to evaluate pleural space.
- Useful in determining etiology of pleural effusion.
- Useful for evaluation of loculated effusion or emphysema.

Treatment: A diagnostic thoracentesis may be performed to determine underlying disease process. Treatment may vary depending on the cause of the pleural effusion.

Prognosis: Depends on the cause, course of treatment, and other health-related issues involving the patient.

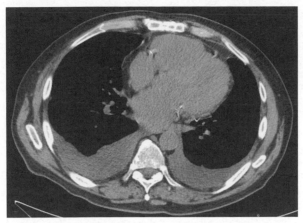

FIGURE 1. **Pleural Effusion.** CT with soft tissue windows shows fluid within the dependent pleural space bilaterally.

Pulmonary Emboli

Description: A pulmonary emboli (PE) is an obstruction of the pulmonary artery or one of its branches by an embolus.

Etiology: Generally results from dislodged thrombi originating in the leg veins. Risk factors include long-term immobility, chronic pulmonary disease, congestive heart failure, recent surgery, advanced age, pregnancy, fractures or surgery to the lower extremities, burns, obesity, malignancy, and use of oral contraceptives.

Epidemiology: This is the most common pulmonary complication in hospitalized patients. The incidence rate of new cases is between 600,000 and 700,000 annually with 100,000 to 200,000 deaths. Men and women are equally affected. Advancing age increases risk of developing pulmonary emboli.

Signs and Symptoms: Chest pain, shortness of breath, hemoptysis (coughing of blood), and swelling of legs.

Imaging Characteristics: Spiral CT pulmonary angiography (CTPA) is the best noninvasive test for diagnosing (PE) and is gradually replacing the V/Q lung scan. CT is reliable in diagnosing emboli in larger central pulmonary arteries but may miss small emboli in smaller subsegmental peripheral pulmonary arteries which may not be clinically significant.

CT
- IV contrast study demonstrates a hypodense plug-like structure within the pulmonary artery.
- Filling defects in the pulmonary arteries.
- Obstruction of the pulmonary arteries.
- Combined CTPA and CT venography (CTV) may show filling defects in the iliac and femoral veins.

Treatment: Depending on the size and location of the emboli and the patient's condition, the patient may be treated with oxygen as needed, IV heparin, warfarin, and/or thrombolytic therapy.

Prognosis: Good with early diagnosis and treatment. Large saddle emboli can be fatal.

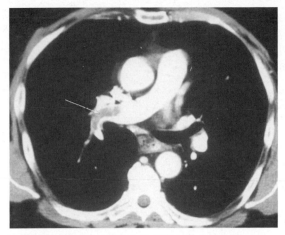

FIGURE 1. Pulmonary Emboli. CTPA shows large filling defect (clot) in the right main pulmonary artery (*arrow*) extending into the lower lobe pulmonary arteries.

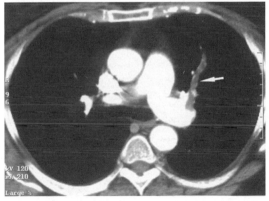

FIGURE 2. Pulmonary Emboli. CTPA shows linear filling defect representing a clot in the left upper lobe pulmonary artery (*arrow*).

Pulmonary Fibrosis

Description: Scarring throughout the lungs which results in a loss of elasticity.

Etiology: There are several possible causes such as pneumoconiosis, histoplasmosis, radiation therapy used to treat chest-related tumors, and unknown (idiopathic pulmonary fibrosis).

Epidemiology: The exact number is unknown. However, for idiopathic pulmonary fibrosis, approximately three to five cases per 100,000 persons are estimated to be affected.

Signs and Symptoms: Shortness of breath, coughing, and reduced tolerance of exercise.

Imaging Characteristics:

CT
- HRCT is best with thin-section imaging (1 mm) and bone windows to evaluate the lung.
- Radiation fibrosis is restricted to the radiation port field.

Treatment: Treatment may be determined based on the specific diagnosis. Basic supportive methods include smoking cessation, oxygen therapy, and immunosuppressive agents. Surgical intervention may be used in select cases.

Prognosis: Varied and depends on the specific etiology and severity of the condition.

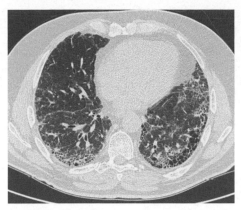

FIGURE 1. Pulmonary Fibrosis. HRCT of the chest shows honeycombing in the peripheral lung bases with associated traction bronchiectasis.

Pulmonary Metastatic Disease

Description: The lung is frequently the site of metastatic disease from primary cancers outside the lung. Metastatic spread to the lung is usually considered to be incurable. A solitary pulmonary lesion may represent a metastasis process or a new primary lung cancer.

Etiology: The lungs are the most frequent site of metastatic spread. Metastatic spread is accomplished through the blood circulation or lymphatic system.

Epidemiology: Carcinoma of the kidney, breast, pancreas, colon, and uterus are the most likely to metastasize to the lungs.

Signs and Symptoms: The most common symptom is a cough. Other related symptoms include hemoptysis, wheezing, fever, dyspnea, and chest pain.

Imaging Characteristics: CT is the modality of choice for imaging pulmonary metastatic disease.

CT
- Typically shows multiple bilateral lung masses that are noncalcified.
- May also show mediastinal lymphadenopathy.

Treatment: Surgical resection when possible. Radiation therapy may be used when tumors are inoperable, and chemotherapy for palliative use.

Prognosis: Poor.

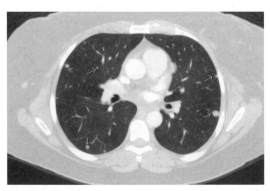

FIGURE 1. **Pulmonary Metastatic Disease.** Multiple peripheral pulmonary metastases (*arrows*).

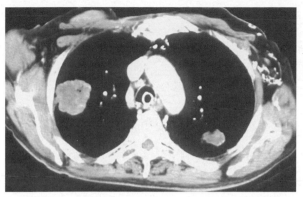

FIGURE 2. **Pulmonary Metastatic Disease.** CT of the chest with mediastinal windows demonstrating bilateral upper lobe masses with areas of low density representing necrosis.

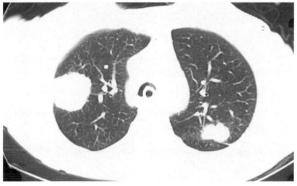

FIGURE 3. **Pulmonary Metastatic Disease.** CT with lung window showing bilateral upper lobe masses with slightly irregular margins consistent with metastatic lesions.

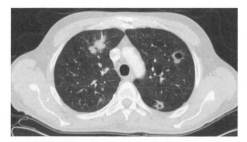

FIGURE 4. **Pulmonary Metastatic Disease.**
Multiple solid and cavitary pulmonary metastases in a patient with known squamous cell carcinoma.

Sarcoidosis

Description: This multisystem disease primarily affects the lungs and intrathoracic lymph nodes.

Etiology: Unknown.

Epidemiology: Affects African Americans more than Caucasians. Males are affected 2:1 more than females. Average age is between 25 and 35 years.

Signs and Symptoms: Dyspnea during activity, cough, and chest pain occur in many cases. Hemoptysis may be rare.

Imaging Characteristics:

CT
- HRCT is best method to evaluate lung parenchyma.
- Hilar and mediastinal lymphadenopathy most common intrathoracic manifestation.
- Noncaseating granulomas present as multiple, round, mass-like consolidations.

Treatment: Corticosteroids are often used. Lung transplantation may be considered for advanced disease.

Prognosis: Patients with pulmonary lesions and impaired function may have poorer outcome.

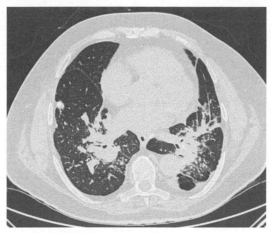

FIGURE 1. Sarcoidosis. HRCT shows increased opacification predominately involving the mid lung with peripheral nodules and atelectasis in the middle lobe and lingual.

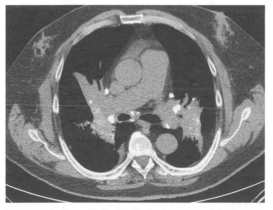

FIGURE 2. Sarcoidosis. Mediastinal windows show densely calcified mediastinal and hilar lymph nodes consistent with sarcoid.

MEDIASTINUM

Hodgkin Disease

Description: Hodgkin disease is a primary neoplastic malignancy of the lymphatic system. It is characterized by painless enlargement of the lymph nodes, spleen, and other lymphatic tissues. Histological evaluation is made upon identifying the classic Reed-Sternberg cell.

Etiology: The exact cause is unknown; however, the Epstein-Barr virus is a possible etiologic agent.

Epidemiology: Hodgkin disease accounts for less than 1% of all malignancies and 14% of all malignant lymphomas. There is a bimodal age distribution. The first peak occurs between 15 and 35 years of age and the second between 55 and 75 years. This malignancy occurs more often in males than females.

Signs and Symptoms: Patients may experience painless, palpable lymph node(s), dry cough, weight loss (>10%), fever, and night sweats.

Imaging Characteristics: CT is the preferred modality to diagnosis mediastinal and retroperitoneal lymphadenopathy.

CT
- Enlarged mediastinal lymph nodes.
- Enlarged retroperitoneal and mesenteric lymph nodes.
- Enlarged spleen and liver.

Treatment: Radiation therapy may be used to administer a tumoricidal dose, chemotherapy is used typically with a combined multidrug regimen, and surgery is usually used for biopsy purposes only or for splenectomy.

Prognosis: Generally good with early diagnosis and treatment.

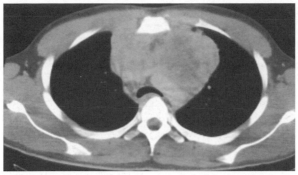

FIGURE 1. **Hodgkin Disease.** Contrast-enhanced CT shows a very large anterior mediastinal mass displacing the aortic arch posteriorly and compressing the trachea. This mediastinal mass in this young patient is consistent with lymphoma or Hodgkin disease.

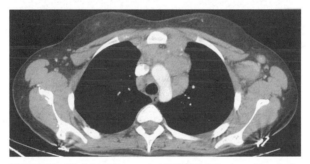

FIGURE 2. **Hodgkin Disease.** Axial CECT of the chest shows bulky anterior mediastinal and left axillary lymphadenopathy in this patient with Hodgkin lymphoma.

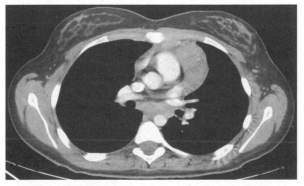

FIGURE 3. **Hodgkin Disease.** Axial CECT of the chest shows the congolomeration of nodes extending down and appearing as an anterior mediastinal mass.

Thymoma

Description: Cancer of the thymus.

Etiology: Unknown; however, this cancer originates from the epithelial cells of the thymus.

Epidemiology: This accounts for approximately 20% of all mediastinal tumors and the most common primary tumor of the anterior mediastinum. Thymomas occur 75% of the time in the anterior mediastinum, 15% in both anterior and superior mediastina, and 6% in the superior mediastina, and the remainder occur either ectopically or in the posterior mediastinum. The peak incidence of thymoma is between the fourth and fifth decades of life. Males and females are equally affected.

Signs and Symptoms: About one-third are asymptomatic, another one-third present with symptoms related to encroachment on surrounding structures such as cough, chest pain, superior vena cava syndrome, dysphagia, and hoarseness due to laryngeal nerve involvement. Another one-third is found incidentally during radiographic examinations for myasthenia gravis (MG).

Imaging Characteristics:

CT
- Typically seen as smooth or lobulated masses 5 to 10 cm in size.
- IV contrast examination is good to show relationship between tumor mass and surrounding vascular structures, degree of vascularity, and other anatomical-related structures.
- Calcification may be seen.
- Invasive involvement seen as (1) poorly defined or infiltrative margins; (2) definite vascular or chest wall invasion; (3) irregular interface with adjacent; and (4) evidence of spread to pleura.

MRI
- Typically seen as smooth or lobulated masses 5 to 10 cm in size.
- T1-weighted (T1W) images of tumor are low to intermediate signal similar to skeletal muscle.
- T2-weighted appear with high signal.
- About one-third appear with mixed (heterogeneous) signal due to the tumor being comprised of necrosis, hemorrhage, and cystic changes.
- Invasive involvement seen as (1) poorly defined or infiltrative margins; (2) definite vascular or chest wall invasion; (3) irregular interface with adjacent; and (4) evidence of spread to pleura.

Treatment: Surgical intervention for initial treatment. Adjuvant radiation therapy may be used in complete or incomplete resection of the tumor. Chemotherapy may be used for invasive and metastasized cases.

Prognosis: Better prognosis when detected early. Prognosis is worse when tumor is invasive or has metastasized.

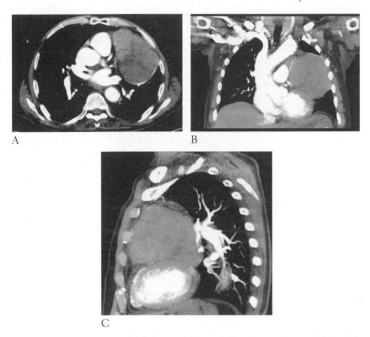

FIGURE 1. Thymoma. Axial (A), coronal MPR (B), and sagittal MPR (C) CECT images show a large lobulated mass within the left anterior mediastinum. This was found to be a mixed lymphoepithelial thymoma at surgery.

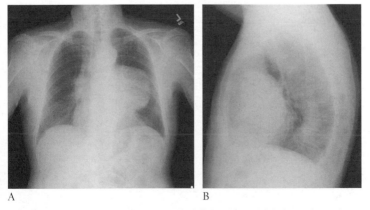

FIGURE 2. Thymoma. Posteroanterior (PA) (A) and lateral (B) chest radiographs show a large left anterior mediastinal mass projecting over the left lung.

AORTA

Aortic Coarctation

Description: Is a localized abnormal narrowing of the descending (usually upper thoracic) aorta. Other cardiovascular abnormalities (e.g., bicuspid aortic valve) may be present.

Etiology: This is a congenital heart defect.

Epidemiology: About 6% to 8% of all congenital heart defects. The majority (approximately 80%) of cases are detected in young children.

Signs and Symptoms: Neonates and infants may show tachypnea, tachycardia, and difficult breathing. Additional signs will show differences in blood pressure between upper and lower extremities and reduced or absent pulse in the lower extremities. Hypertension or murmur may be seen in younger children. In older children and adults, differences in blood pressure measurements between the upper extremities and one leg may occur.

Imaging Characteristics:

CT
- CTA with MPR, maximum intensity projection (MIP), and 3D images are helpful.

MRI
- CMR is most effective in showing anatomy and physiology of the aortic arch.
- CMR good in postsurgical patients.

Treatment: Surgery.

Prognosis: Depends on several factors; however, this lifelong condition has a guarded prognosis mostly associated with other cardiovascular complications and possible reoccurrence.

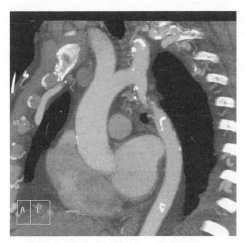

FIGURE 1. Aortic Coarctation. CTA sagittal oblique MPR of the chest shows severe narrowing in a different patient.

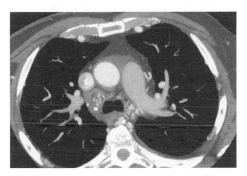

FIGURE 2. Aortic Coarctation. CTA axial of the chest at the level of the severe narrowing in the same patient as Figure 1 shows multiple collaterals and enlarged intercostal arteries with rib notching.

Aortic Dissection

Description: An aortic dissection occurs when blood enters into the wall of the artery dissecting between the layers and creating a cavity or false lumen in the vessel wall. Dissecting aneurysms are classified into two types according to the Stanford classification scale. Dissecting aneurysms involving the ascending aorta are classified as Type A. Those involving only the descending aorta are Type B.

Etiology: Most likely result from a tearing of the wall of the artery.

Epidemiology: The peak incidence occurs in the sixth and seventh decades of life. Males are more commonly affected than females. Approximately 60% of dissecting aneurysms are Type A and 40% are Type B. The most common predisposing condition is hypertension. Other predisposing factors include Marfan syndrome, coarctation, bicuspid aortic valve, aortitis, and pregnancy. Aortic dissection may be iatrogenic and result at the site of an aortic cannulation, bypass grafting, cross-clamping, or during a catheterization procedure.

Signs and Symptoms: Patients may present with pain in the chest or abdomen. Approximately 15% to 20% of patients present asymptomatic.

Imaging Characteristics: CT with IV contrast is the best (readily available and faster) imaging modality for the evaluation of aortic dissection.

CT
- Precontrast images may show enlarged aorta, intimal flap, and intimal calcification.
- Precontrast images show the thrombosed false lumen with a higher attenuation value.
- Precontrast images show pericardial, mediastinal, and/or pleural hemorrhage as secondary to rupture.
- Postcontrast images show contrast-filled true and false lumens separated by the intimal flap.
- Postcontrast images show a delayed enhancement of the false lumen.
- Postcontrast images show compression of the true lumen by the thrombosed false lumen.
- Postcontrast images show ischemia/infarction or organs supplied by vessels branching from the false lumen.

MRI
- Good for the evaluation of an aortic dissection.
- MRI/MRA offers multiplanar imaging and no need for IV contrast.
- Shows same findings as CT.

Treatment: Depends on the type (Stanford classification) of dissecting aneurysm. Type A dissections, those involving the ascending aorta, usually require surgery. Type B dissecting aneurysms are usually managed medically to control hypertension.

Prognosis: Good with Type B dissection. If untreated, Type A dissection has a high mortality and may result in cardiac tamponade.

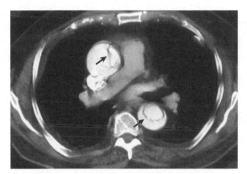

FIGURE 1. Type A Dissecting Aneurysm. Axial CT with IV contrast demonstrates a Type A aortic dissecting aneurysm involving both the ascending and descending thoracic aorta showing a double lumen separated by the intimal flap.

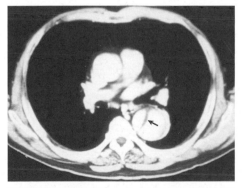

FIGURE 2. Type B Dissecting Aneurysm. Axial CT with IV contrast shows a Type B dissecting aneurysm involving the descending thoracic aorta with two lumens (true and false) separated by an intimal flap.

BREAST

Breast Cancer

Description: Cancer of the breast. There are several different types of breast cancer. Ductal carcinoma in situ (DCIS) is also known as intraductal carcinoma. DCIS is the most common type of noninvasive breast cancer. Lobular carcinoma in situ (LCIS) is known also as lobular neoplasm. LCIS is a type of noninvasive breast cancer; however, it may become invasive. Invasive or infiltrating ductal carcinoma (IDC) spreads through the lymphatic system and blood stream. Invasive or infiltrating lobular carcinoma (ILC) can also metastasize throughout the body.

Etiology: A variety of risk factors (e.g., family history, age, reproductive history, use of oral contraceptives, and lifestyle) may increase chances of developing breast cancer.

Epidemiology: DCIS accounts for one in five of new breast cancers detected. IDC accounts for about 8 out of 10 invasive breast cancers. ILC represents a smaller number of invasive breast cancers. About 99% of all breast cancers affect females.

Imaging Characteristics: Mammography used for screening.

CT
- May be detected as an incidental finding.
- Useful for staging and radiation therapy treatment planning.

MRI
- Contrast-enhanced MRI useful in detecting and characterizing benign and malignant breast diseases.
- Fat saturation techniques useful in suppressing the signal from fat tissue.

Treatment: Depending on the type of breast cancer and stage, surgery intervention, radiation therapy, and chemotherapy may be used.

Prognosis: Depends on the type of breast cancer and stage.

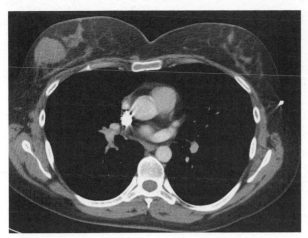

FIGURE 1. **Breast Cancer.** CECT shows a soft-tissue mass in the right breast consistent with breast cancer.

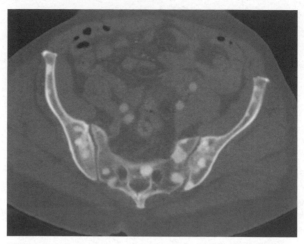

FIGURE 2. Breast Cancer. CECT with bone windows shows
multiple osteoblastic breast cancer metastases within the sacrum and
iliac wings.

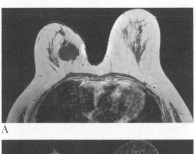

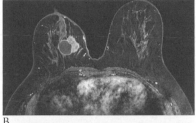

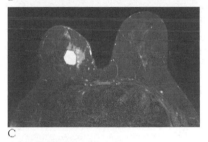

RIGHT BREAST
1 Finding, Total Angio Volume 37.5

Finding R1

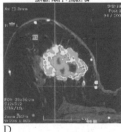

R, UI, 2 o'clock, middle

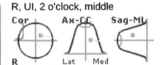

Diameters: 5.5 x 3.5 x 5.8 cm
Angio Volume: 37.5 cc

FIGURE 3. Breast Cancer. T1W MR (A) shows a large 5-cm spiculated mass in the right breast. T1W fat-suppressed postcontrast MR image (B) demonstrates enhancement of the solid component. T2W image (C) shows a hyperintense 3-cm fluid collection next to the breast cancer which may represent a mucinous or necrotic component. In image (D), computer-assisted detection software characterizes the enhancement kinetics of the mass.

Breast Implant Leakage

Description: Silicone gel-filled breast implants were first used in patients in the early 1960s. Initially, silicone exposure was thought to represent a health risk to women with breast implants. To date, however, scientific evidence supporting an association between silicone gel-filled breast implants and classic autoimmune disease is unclear. Virtually all silicone gel-filled breast implants "bleed" small amounts of silicone fluid through the intact implant shell. This is not to be confused with larger amounts of "leakage" of silicone gel caused by a rupture in the structural integrity of the implant shell.

Etiology: Causes for implant leakage (i.e., bleeding or rupture) are unclear, but possibilities include upper body exercise and activity, submuscular placement, trauma, mammography, and weak implant wall design.

Epidemiology: In 1999, there were an estimated 2 million women with breast implants in the United States. The absolute rupture rate of implants in the general population of all implant patients has yet to be measured. Reported implant rupture rates for patients seen for known or suspected problems have ranged anywhere from 22.9% to 92%.

Signs and Symptoms: Patients with breast implant silicone gel leakage may be asymptomatic.

Imaging Characteristics: MRI is useful in the evaluation of the breast implant. The fluid in breast implants appears with similar signal intensities as cerebrospinal fluid.

MRI

- Good for evaluating the integrity of the breast implant (e.g., intact, herniation, partially or complete rupture, intracapsular and extracapsular).
- With extracapsular rupture MRI shows collection of silicone outside the implant lumen.
- Intracapsular rupture demonstrates multiple curvilinear low-signal intensity lines commonly referred to as the linguine sign is seen within the high-signal silicone gel.

Treatment: Surgical removal of ruptured implants and evacuation of silicone or polyurethane when possible.

Prognosis: Postsurgical prognosis should be good, barring unforeseen complications.

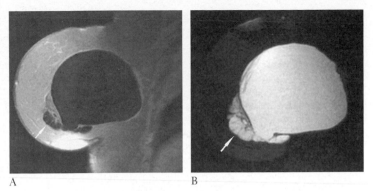

A   B

FIGURE 1. **Rupture of Breast Implant.** T1-weighted (A) and T2-weighted (B) MR images of the breast show collections of silicone (*arrows*) outside the implant lumen that are diagnostic of extracapsular rupture.

TRAUMA

Aortic Tear

Description: An aortic tear involves a traumatic tearing or laceration of the aorta.

Etiology: The majority of these cases are associated with high-speed motor vehicle (deceleration) accidents. Others may occur as a result of falls, crushing injuries, or blast-related (compression) injuries.

Epidemiology: Over 90% of aortic tears occur at the aortic isthmus (just distal to the origin of the left subclavian artery). This is the site where the ligamentum arteriosum attaches to the aortic arch and the pulmonary artery.

Signs and Symptoms: Many patients do not demonstrate any visible external signs of chest trauma. However, as a result of head trauma, a great number of these patients present with altered mental status. In patients with a history involving a rapid deceleration, the possibility of an aortic injury is suspected.

Imaging Characteristics:

CT
- A mediastinal hematoma occurs in association with the tear.
- Loss of normal contour of the aorta at the site of the tear.
- Extravasation of contrast.
- Periaortic hematoma.
- Small aortic tears may be difficult to visualize.

Treatment: Emergency surgical intervention.

Prognosis: Eighty percent to 90% of all patients with aortic laceration/tear die at the scene of the accident or are dead on arrival at the hospital. For the 10% to 20% of the patients that arrive at the hospital alive, a rapid diagnosis and surgical repair can produce survival rates. However, other injuries related to the initial traumatic event may complicate the patient's recovery.

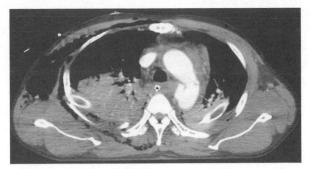

FIGURE 1. **Aortic Tear.** Axial CECT shows a contour irregularity of the aortic arch with small intraluminal linear filling defects and pseudoaneurysm.

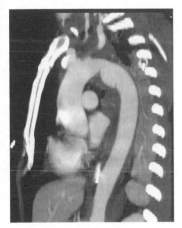

FIGURE 2. **Aortic Tear.** CTA sagittal oblique MPR shows irregular aortic contour just distal to the ductus arterious due to traumatic aortic laceration.

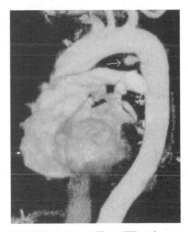

FIGURE 3. **Aortic Tear.** CTA volume rendered (VR) in a different patient, shows a posttraumatic pseudoaneurysm (*arrow*).

Diaphragmatic Hernia

Description: A congenital diaphragmatic hernia is an abnormal protrusion of some abdominal contents (e.g., fat, stomach, loop of bowel) through an opening in the diaphragm into the chest cavity. There are three common sites of herniation: (1) anterior parasternal hiatus (foramen of Morgagni); (2) esophageal hiatus; and (3) posterior pleuroperitoneal hiatus (foramen of Bochdalek). In infants, the most common site of herniation is through the foramen of Bochdalek. Diaphragmatic hernias are most common on the left side.

Etiology: Congenital or acquired.

Epidemiology: Incident rate of approximately 1 in every 2000 to 3000 live births and represents about 8% of all major congenital anomalies. Occurs equally in males and females.

Signs and Symptoms: Difficulty in breathing is most common symptom. Bluish color of skin and tachycardia may also be seen.

Imaging Characteristics: Chest x-ray is usually diagnostic.

CT
- Shows middle mediastinal mass in lower thorax.
- Shows air or contrast within the hernia.
- MPRs are helpful in showing abdominal structures in the chest cavity.
- MPRs useful for surgical planning.

Treatment: Emergency surgical repair is required.

Prognosis: Depending on lung development, there is a good outcome expected.

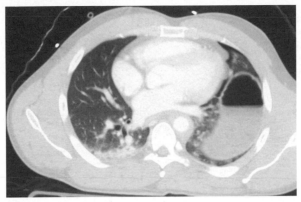

FIGURE 1. Diaphragmatic Hernia. CECT shows the stomach within the left chest at the level of the heart. There is also a small left anterior pneumothorax in the trauma patient.

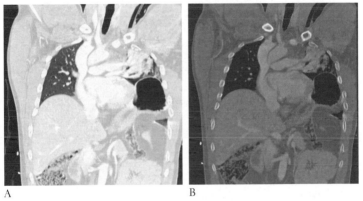

A   B

FIGURE 2. Diaphragmatic Hernia. CECT coronal MPRs with lung window (A) and soft tissue windows (B) show the stomach herniating through a defect in the diaphragm into the left chest.

Lung Contusion

Description: Bruise to the lung.

Etiology: Caused by severe (blunt or penetrating) trauma to the chest.

Epidemiology: Most thoracic trauma is the result of motor vehicle accidents. Approximately 20% to 25% of deaths are related to thoracic injury.

Signs and Symptoms: Difficulty in breathing, chest pain, and cough. Fractures to the ribs and sternum are common. Coughing up blood, excessive sweating, fainting, and confusion may occur in severe cases.

Imaging Characteristics:

CT
- Useful in evaluating the thoracic cavity for bony fractures.
- Useful in evaluating the lungs and thorax for trauma-related injuries such as pneumothorax, hemothorax, acute respiratory distress syndrome (ARDS), pleural effusion, and subcutaneous emphysema.

Treatment: Stabilize the patient with IV fluids, oxygen therapy, and pain medication. Surgical intervention may be required.

Prognosis: Depends on the severity of the injury and other underlying conditions.

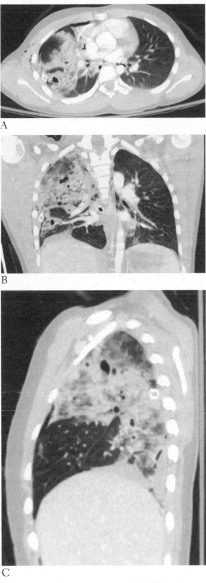

FIGURE 1. Lung Contusion. CECT axial (A), coronal MPR (B), and sagittal MPR (C) images of a trauma patient showing the extensive pulmonary contusion of the right upper and lower lobes. There is confluent lung opacification with multiple small posttraumatic pneumatoceles.

Pneumothorax

Description: A pneumothorax is a collection of air within the pleural cavity.

Etiology: Primarily results from traumatic blunt injury to the chest.

Epidemiology: A pneumothorax occurs in up to 40% of patients experiencing blunt trauma to the chest. It may be associated with or without rib fractures. A laceration of the visceral pleura from a rib fracture is seen in approximately 70% of cases. Young males in their second to fourth decades are more commonly affected.

Signs and Symptoms: The patient presents with chest pain and dyspnea.

Imaging Characteristics: Plain x-ray is the primary choice for detecting and evaluating a pneumothorax. CT is useful in evaluating difficult cases such as a small pneumothorax in the supine patient.

CT
- A collection of fluid and air is seen within the pleural cavity.
- Rib fractures may be seen penetrating into the chest.
- Lung contusions or lacerations may be seen.
- Associated abnormal injuries may be seen.

Treatment: A thoracostomy (chest) tube may be inserted to reexpand the lung. Surgical intervention may be required in severe cases.

Prognosis: Depends on the extent of the pneumothorax and other associated injuries. A good recovery should be expected.

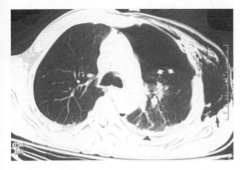

FIGURE 1. Pneumothorax. Contrast CT of the chest shows large left pneumothorax with air outlining the visceral pleura (*short arrows*). There is minimal hemothorax (*arrowhead*). There is a large subcutaneous emphysema (*long arrows*) of the left chest wall.

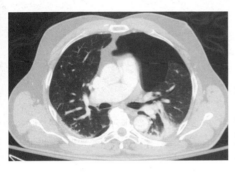

FIGURE 2. Pneumothorax. Axial CECT of the chest shows a large left pneumothorax as abnormal air density within the pleural space and a partially collapsed left lung.

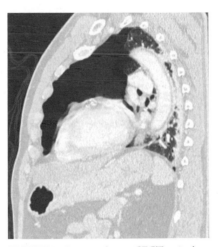

FIGURE 3. Pneumothorax. CECT sagittal MPR of the same patient shows a large left anterior pneumothorax.

PART VI

Abdomen

GASTROINTESTINAL

Carcinoid

Description: Carcinoids are rare, slow-growing cancers which start in the lining of the gastrointestinal tract.

Etiology: Unknown; however, genetic involvement is suspected.

Epidemiology: Overall, 1.5 cases per 100,000 population. They occur mostly in the appendix (50%) and small bowel (20%). The ileum is the most frequent site of involvement in the small bowel. Females and older adults are more commonly affected.

Signs and Symptoms: The signs and symptoms may be vague. Patients may experience abdominal pain, bleeding, and bowel obstruction.

Imaging Characteristics: Primary tumors may be small. Aggressive tumors >2 cm may have a necrotic center. May mimic a lymphoma.

CT
- Appear as a bright wall mass with IV contrast.
- Thick fibrotic stranding radiates from the mass to adjacent bowel.
- Usually metastasize to the liver, are hypervascular, and best seen on the arterial phase.

MRI
- T1-weighted signal is isointense to muscle.
- T1-weighted postgadolinium shows bright signal on delayed studies.
- T2-weighted signal may vary from isointense to hyperintense to muscle.

Treatment: Surgery is the treatment of choice. Chemotherapy is helpful for metastatic spread.

Prognosis: Results are better if complete resection of the localized tumor is accomplished.

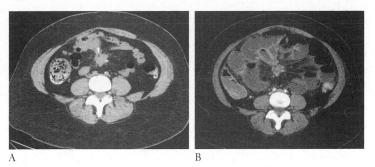

A   B

FIGURE 1. **Carcinoid.** Pre- (A) and postcontrast (B) CTs of the abdomen show an enhancing, partially calcified, stellate mid-abdominal mesenteric mass with radiating bands of fibrosis and retraction of the surrounding small bowel, giving a classic "sunburst" appearance.

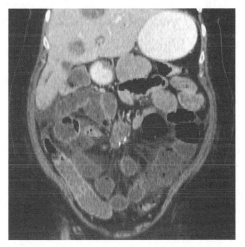

FIGURE 2. **Carcinoid.** Contrast-enhanced CT (CECT) coronal multiplanar reconstruction (MPR) image shows similar findings as the axial images. In this image, multiple low-attenuation liver metastases can be seen.

Colorectal Cancer

Description: Colorectal cancer (adenocarcinoma of the colon) is the most common malignant tumor affecting the gastrointestinal tract. Colorectal cancer often begins as a polyp which may become malignant if left untreated.

Etiology: A number of factors such as heredity, inflammatory bowel disease (e.g., ulcerative colitis and Crohn's disease), physical inactivity, overweight and obesity, diabetes, diet, smoking, and alcohol intake are thought to play a role in the development of colorectal cancer.

Epidemiology: Colorectal cancer is the third leading cause of cancer death for men and women in the United States. African Americans have a higher incidence rate than white people, while Hispanics/Latinos, American Indians, and Alaska natives have a lower incidence rate. Male are slightly more affected than females. Incidence and death rates increase in individuals 50 years and older.

Signs and Symptoms: In its early stage, colorectal cancer is often asymptomatic. Patients may experience rectal bleeding, blood in the stool, cramping lower abdominal pain, change in bowel habits, and new onset of constipation.

Imaging Characteristics: Primary tumor may be a colon polyp usually >1 cm. Polyps may appear as a sessile or pedunculated mass arising from the bowel wall and protruding into the lumen.

CT
- Chest, abdomen, and pelvic scan for staging purposes.
- Central low attenuation represents hemorrhage or necrosis.
- Air within the tumor may indicate ulceration.
- Regional lymph nodes >1 cm are considered positive for metastatic spread.
- Distant metastatic spread is mostly seen in the liver (75%), lung (5% to 50%), adrenal gland (14%), and elsewhere.
- Thin-section imaging is required for CT colonography.
- Fecal and fluid tagging is beneficial in CT colonography.

MRI
- Normal colon has a thin wall with haustrations, and enhances minimally with IV contrast.
- T2-weighted single-shot echo-train spin-echo and True-FISP help control for bowel motion.

- IV contrast-enhanced with fat suppression T1-weighted-spoiled gradient echo or 3D gradient echo is helpful in evaluating the colon.
- Dark-lumen technique may show a polyp protruding into the lumen.
- Endorectal MR may be helpful in evaluating the rectum.

Treatment: Depending on the stage of the cancer, surgery, chemotherapy, and radiation therapy may be used.

Prognosis: Colon screening is beneficial in early detection and treatment. The 5-year survival for colorectal cancer (including all stages) is about 65%.

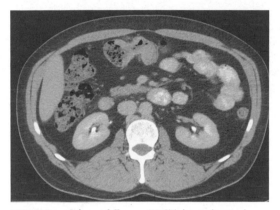

FIGURE 1. **Colorectal Cancer.** CECT shows abnormal mural thickening of the mid transverse colon with luminal narrowing and surrounding soft-tissue bands extending into the surrounding fat which likely represents extracolonic tumor extension.

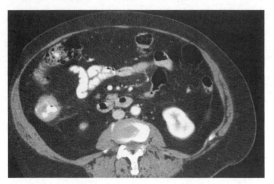

FIGURE 2. **Colorectal Cancer.** CECT with positive oral contrast shows abnormal mural thickening of the right hemicolon.

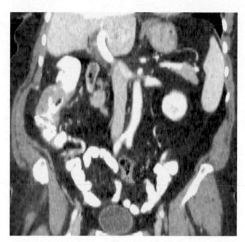

FIGURE 3. **Colorectal Cancer.** CECT coronal MPR image shows a several centimeter segment of thickened bowel wall involving the mid-right colon. This is typical of colon cancer.

Crohn's Disease

Description: Crohn's disease is an inflammatory condition which can affect any part of the alimentary tract. However, the small bowel, specifically the terminal ileum, is most commonly affected.

Etiology: Though the precise cause remains unknown, there seems to be a combination of genetic, immunologic, and infectious factors involved.

Epidemiology: Crohn's disease can occur at any age; however, the disease usually presents in adolescents and young adults between the ages of 15 and 35 years. It has a bimodal distribution with the first peak being in the teens and twenties and the second peak occurring in the fifties through the seventies.

Signs and Symptoms: Patients present with persistent or recurrent diarrhea, abdominal pain with cramps, weight loss, and fever.

Imaging Characteristics: Key characteristics include: (1) bowel wall thickening greater than 1 cm; (2) involvement of >15 cm bowel; and (3) mural enhancement.

CT
- IV contrast shows marked bowel wall enhancement.
- Fistula may be seen.
- Mesenteric inflammation is seen as diffuse haziness and increased density in the mesenteric fat.
- Normal bowel "skip areas" may be seen between diseased segments of bowel.

MRI
- T2-weighted single-shot echo-train spin-echo and IV gadolinium-enhanced T1-weighted with fat suppression spoiled gradient echo demonstrates dilated bowel and inflammatory changes.
- 3D gradient echo demonstrates characteristic findings: mural enhancement, skip lesions (patchy areas of inflammation), and mesenteric inflammatory changes.

Treatment: Is focused on reducing the inflammation and maintaining good nutrition.

Prognosis: There is no cure for this disease. Patients with Crohn's disease are at an increased risk for colorectal cancer.

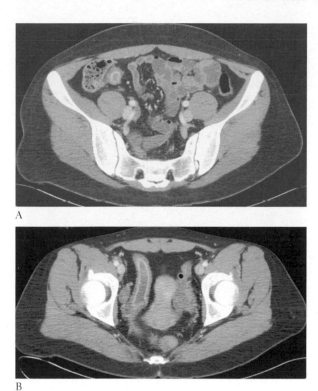

A

B

FIGURE 1. **Crohn's Disease.** CECT axial images (A, B) show intense enhancement of the mucosa and low-attenuation edematous thickened submucosa of the terminal ileum consistent with Crohn's disease.

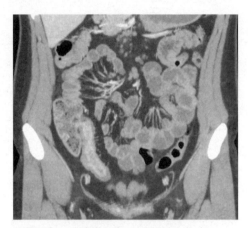

FIGURE 2. **Crohn's Disease.** CECT coronal
MPR image in the same patient shows mesenteric
hypervascularity ("comb sign") and proliferation of the
adjacent mesenteric fat.

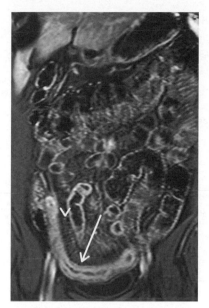

FIGURE 3. **Crohn's Disease.** Postcontrast
T1W fat saturation MR image (e-THRIVE)
shows an enhancing thickened long segment
terminal ileum (*arrow*) as well as a "comb
sign" with mesenteric hypervascularity
(*arrowhead*).

Free Intraperitoneal Air

Description: Free air in the peritoneal cavity, also known as a pneumo-peritoneum, is a collection of air or gas in the peritoneal cavity.

Etiology: This condition can be the result of several factors such as iatrogenic perforation (e.g., laparoscopy, leaking surgical anastomosis, enema tip), disease process (e.g., ulcer, ingested foreign body, ruptured intestine), and penetrating trauma. The most common cause is a perforated ulcer.

Epidemiology: It may occur in anyone who has experienced any of the above-listed factors.

Signs and Symptoms: Pain and tenderness usually result from a perforation of the bowel.

Imaging Characteristics: Best detected on lung windows (WL = −400 to −600; WW = 1000 to 2000).

CT
- Gold standard for detection of a pneumoperitoneum.
- IV contrast may not be required.
- Oral contrast (water soluble) may be used to better visualize the GI tract and to demonstrate a leak in the bowel.
- Appears hypodense.
- Free air is classified according to the anatomical location.
- Scanning in the decubitus position will assist in interpreting difficult cases.

Treatment: Depends on the etiology.

Prognosis: Depends on the etiology.

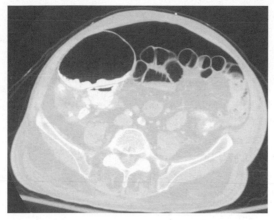

FIGURE 1. Free Intraperitoneal Air. Axial CT shows a large amount of intra-abdominal free air outlining multiple loops of bowel.

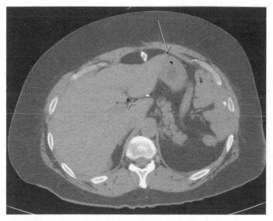

FIGURE 2. Free Intraperitoneal Air. Axial CT demonstrating less dramatic example of extraluminal intra-abdominal free air (*arrows*) in a patient with a duodenal perforation.

Gastric Carcinoma

Description: Gastric (adenocarcinoma) carcinoma is one of the most common cancers in the world. Adenocarcinomas make up approximately 95% of all malignant cancers affecting the stomach.

Etiology: Dietary and environmental factors may influence the onset of the cancer. Nitrates, pickled foods, salted fish and meat products, and smoked foods have been associated with gastric carcinoma. Cigarette smoking increases the risk of developing gastric carcinoma.

Epidemiology: Approximately 21,000 cases detected, with about 10,500 deaths annually. More commonly affects those 65 years and older, with an average age of 70. Males are slightly higher at risk than females.

Signs and Symptoms: Asymptomatic in early stages. Epigastric pain, bloating, nausea and vomiting, dysphagia (difficulty in swallowing), anorexia (loss of appetite), weight loss, upper GI bleeding (hematemesis), and positive fecal occult blood tests are present.

Imaging Characteristics:

CT
- Primary tumor appears as focal, nodular, or irregular thickening of the gastric wall, or as a polypoid, soft-tissue density, intraluminal mass.
- Dynamic scanning with water ingestion improves detection.
- An advanced cancer shows polyp-type mass with or without ulceration.
- Use of spiral CT with water ingestion and prone position improves tumor detectability.
- Useful for staging.

MRI
- Fast-imaging techniques with breath-holding provides good-quality images.
- Comparable to CT for tumor and node staging.

Treatment: Complete resection of the gastric tumor and involved lymph nodes is the only known possible curative treatment.

Prognosis: Depends on the stage of the cancer. Early stage can have a 5-year survival rate of up to 70%. In advanced stage, the 5-year survival rate is worse.

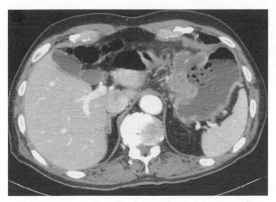

FIGURE 1. **Gastric Carcinoma.** CECT image shows an enhancing, lobulated mass involving the lesser curvature of the stomach with ulceration consistent with gastric carcinoma.

Intussusception

Description: Intussusception is a telescoping (invagination) of one portion of the bowel into another. It is the most common cause of intestinal tract obstruction in pediatrics.

Etiology: It is idiopathic in 90% of the cases involving pediatrics.

Epidemiology: Approximately 95% of cases occur in young children, the remaining occur in adults.

Signs and Symptoms: In infants, a triad of colicky abdominal pain, vomiting, and redcurrant jelly stools may be seen.

Imaging Characteristics:

CT and MRI
- Appears as a bowel-within-bowel configuration.
- Short (3.5 cm) intussusceptions are usually benign.
- Long intussusceptions may involve a pathologic lesion.

Treatment: Hydrostatic barium enema is used to reduce the intussusception in most cases. Surgery is used in the remaining cases.

Prognosis: If untreated, this condition is fatal within a few days.

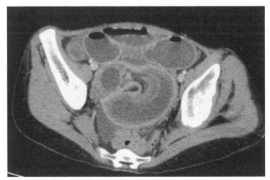

FIGURE 1. **Intussusception.** CECT axial image of the abdomen shows an ileal intussusception resulting in a high-grade proximal obstruction. The axial image shows a "target sign" in the right pelvis as a result of the intussusceptum telescoping into the intussusceptions.

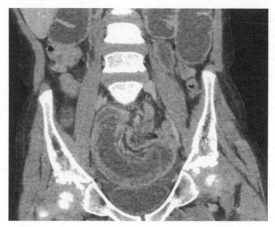

FIGURE 2. **Intussusception.** CECT coronal MPR image shows a sausage-shaped mass in the pelvis with a layered appearance due to alternating enhanced bowel wall and intraluminal fluid.

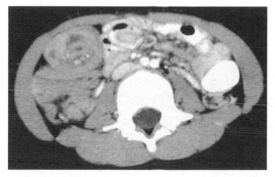

FIGURE 3. **Intussusception.** Ileal-colonic intussusception in a pediatric patient. Axial CECT image shows a classic "target sign" with the terminal ileum surrounded by low-attenuation mesenteric fat within the right colon.

Ischemic Bowel

Description: Ischemic bowel is a disease process which results in a reduced blood flow to the intestinal tract.

Etiology: An insufficient blood flow through the mesenteric vessels is primarily caused by an abnormal fatty/lipid mass within the artery called an atheroma which occludes the vessel. Low cardiac output and trauma may also contribute to this disease. Ischemic bowel may also be caused by embolus.

Epidemiology: Ischemic bowel is primarily seen in an older population. It is rarely seen in individuals younger than 60 years. The average age of the patient when diagnosed is 70 years.

Signs and Symptoms: The patient may present with abdominal pain, tenderness, and bloody diarrhea.

Imaging Characteristics:

CT
- Best modality to diagnose ischemic bowel.
- Poor bowel wall IV contrast enhancement.
- Mesenteric vessel thrombus or vascular engorgement.

MRI
- MR angiography (MRA) is helpful.
- Poor bowel wall IV contrast enhancement.
- Mesenteric vessel thrombus or vascular engorgement.

Treatment: Surgery and interventional procedures such as stenting and balloon angioplasty may be possible methods for treatment.

Prognosis: For transient ischemic attacks, these usually resolve within a few months without any further complications. There is a high mortality rate (90%) associated with occlusive infarct of the mesenteric vessels.

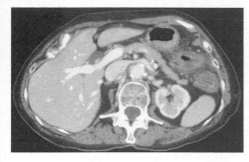

FIGURE 1. Ischemic Bowel. CECT axial image in a different patient shows circumferential wall thickening of the left colon with a "double halo" sign created by the low-attenuation thickened submucosa surrounded by the enhancing mucosal and serosal layers.

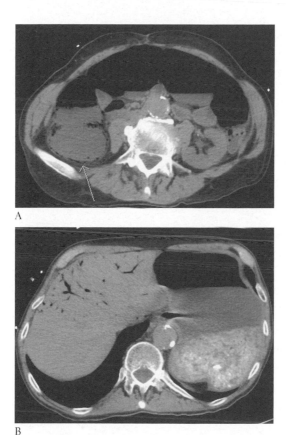

A

B

FIGURE 2. Ischemic Bowel. Nonenhanced CT (NECT) image (A) shows pneumatosis as air within the dependent colon wall on the right (*arrow*). Image (B) shows multiple branching lucencies in the liver extending to the periphery consistent with portal venous gas as a result of ischemic bowel.

Large Bowel Obstruction

Description: Large bowel obstruction (LBO) is a dilation of the colon proximal to an obstructing lesion. This is an emergent situation which requires quick diagnosis and treatment.

Etiology: The majority of LBOs occur as a result of mechanical involvement such as tumors, diverticular disease, or volvulus of the colon. An acute pseudo-obstruction may result from trauma, infections, or cardiac disease.

Epidemiology: The incidence rate for intestinal obstruction is approximately 1 in every 750 people.

Signs and Symptoms: Abdominal distention, abdominal pain, and nausea and vomiting.

Imaging Characteristics: Barium enema or colonoscopy also useful for diagnosis of etiology and level of obstruction.

CT
- Modality of choice for diagnosing LBO particularly for diagnosing obstructing neoplasm, diverticulitis, etc.
- Coronal MPR images are beneficial.
- Air may be seen in dilated bowel.
- Water-soluble contrast should be used if perforation is suspected.

MRI
- Is not routinely indicated—rarely used.
- T2-weighted imaging provides fast, accurate diagnosis of bowel obstruction.

Treatment: Depends on the causative agent. Surgery is frequently indicated. Pseudo-obstruction is treated supportively.

Prognosis: Depends on the causative agent. If detected early, the outcome is better. If secondary to malignancy, the outcome is dependent on the prognosis of the cancer.

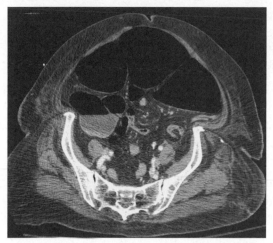

FIGURE 1. **Large Bowel Obstruction.** CECT image shows markedly distended large bowel with an abrupt transition point in the left pelvis due to sigmoid volvulus.

Mesenteric Adenitis

Description: Mesenteric adenitis is a benign inflammation of the mesenteric lymph nodes, usually involving the right lower quadrant (RLQ).

Etiology: Most commonly caused by *Yersinia enterocolitica*, a bacterial infection.

Epidemiology: Less than 8% of patients admitted for appendicitis are discharged with mesenteric adenitis. More commonly affects children 15 years or younger.

Signs and Symptoms: Abdominal pain, fever, diarrhea, and vomiting. These symptoms, in conjunction with the location in the RLQ, often mimic appendicitis.

Imaging Characteristics:

CT
- Enlarged mesenteric lymph nodes (5 mm or greater in size along the short axis of the node) in the right lower quadrant.
- Normal-appearing appendix.
- Bowel wall may or may not be thickened.

Treatment: R/O appendicitis. Antibiotics may be used in moderate to severe cases. Mild cases can be treated with supportive care.

Prognosis: Good, with complete recovery.

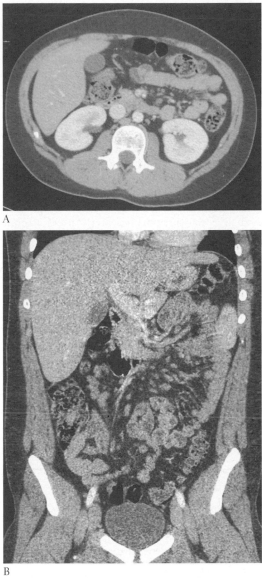

A

B

FIGURE 1. **Mesenteric Adenitis.** CT axial (A) and coronal MPR (B) images show numerous enlarged mesenteric lymph nodes.

Mesenteric Ischemia

Description: Mesenteric or intestinal ischemia is an inadequate blood flow to or from the involved mesenteric (i.e., superior or inferior mesenteric) vessels, which supply a particular section of the small bowel or colon. Further, mesenteric ischemia can be classified as acute or chronic and either arterial or venous in origin.

Etiology: Acute mesenteric ischemia may be the result of an embolus, nonocclusive ischemia, and thrombosis. In the acute form, infarction of the bowel is more common. In the chronic form, bowel viability is not as compromised due to collateral blood flow.

Epidemiology: Arterial ischemia occurs more frequently than venous ischemia. Emboli in the superior mesenteric artery account for about one-third of all acute mesenteric ischemia cases. Nonocclusive ischemia accounts for about one-third of all cases and is due to vasoconstriction episodes. Thrombosis of the mesenteric vessels is the result of atherosclerotic narrowing of the lumen and accounts for about one-third of all cases. This disease usually affects an older population of 60 years or older.

Signs and Symptoms: Most patients will present with a history of nausea, vomiting, and pain.

Imaging Characteristics:

CT
- CTA useful in determining presence or absence of thromboembolism and/or vascular narrowing.
- CTA in arterial phase is useful in evaluating superior and inferior mesenteric vessels.
- Sagittal and coronal MPR, and curved planar reconstruction is helpful in identification of the ischemia.
- CTA on arterial phase will show bowel wall as hypodense for both reversible mesenteric ischemia and infarction.
- CTA during portal or enteral phase will show bowel wall as hypodense for infarction, and near isodense for reversible ischemia.
- Absence of bowel gas.
- Filling defect in vessel with atherosclerosis.

MRI
- 3D contrast-enhanced MR angiography is useful to see narrowing or filling defects in the vessel.

Treatment: Depending on the type and severity of ischemia, surgery, vasodilation, and balloon angioplasty may be used.

Prognosis: If diagnosis and treatment occurs before infarction, mortality is low. If infarction occurs, mortality increases from 70% to 90%.

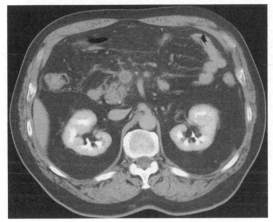

FIGURE 1. **Thrombosis of the Superior Mesenteric Vein.** Axial CECT shows a filling defect within the superior mesenteric vein (SMV) and surrounding "misty mesentery" as a result of venous congestion.

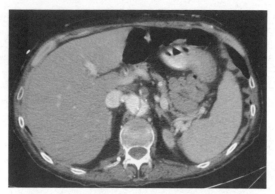

FIGURE 2. **Thrombosis of the Superior Mesenteric Artery.**
Axial CECT shows lack of contrast enhancement within the
superior mesenteric artery (SMA) due to thrombosis.

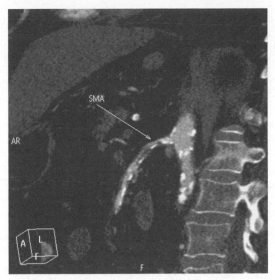

FIGURE 3. **Mesenteric Ischemia.** Sagittal multiplanar reconstruction (MPR) CT image shows dense calcific atherosclerosis of the aorta and SMA. There is a filling defect within the proximal SMA due to thrombosis.

Small Bowel Obstruction

Description: Obstruction of the small bowel is one of the most common causes of abdominal pain.

Etiology: Adhesions that have formed as a result of previous abdominal surgery are the most common cause of small bowel obstruction (SBO). Other extrinsic causes of SBO include malignant tumor, hernia, volvulus, abscess, or hematoma. Intrinsic factors, which occur less frequently, include neoplasm, inflammatory bowel disease, ischemic bowel disease, and intussusception.

Epidemiology: Males and females are equally affected. Small bowel obstruction can occur at any age.

Signs and Symptoms: Obstruction of the bowel typically causes pain, vomiting, distention, and constipation.

Imaging Characteristics: Plain films (supine and upright) are helpful in most cases and should be done first. However, uncertain findings (i.e., false-positive and false-negative studies) occur in as many as 50% of the patients. CT is very accurate in diagnosing SBO (70% to 100%). CT can identify the cause of the obstruction in 50% to 85% of the patients imaged.

CT
- Shows dilated loops of the small bowel (≥ 2.5 cm in diameter).
- Point of transition distal to where the small bowel and colon are collapsed.
- Can diagnose closed loop obstruction (i.e., strangulation), which is usually caused by ischemia and infarction.
- Preferable to use IV contrast. If oral contrast is needed, a water-soluble oral contrast is preferred.

Treatment: Surgical intervention to correct the causative agent.

Prognosis: Depends on the causative agent and other patient-related factors such as the patient's overall health.

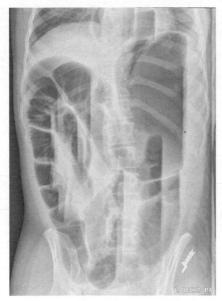

FIGURE 1. **Small Bowel Obstruction.** Left lateral decubitus radiograph of the abdomen shows multiple significantly dilated loops of small bowel with air-fluid levels.

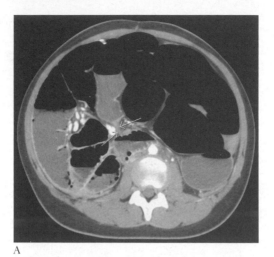

A

FIGURE 2. **Small Bowel Obstruction.** CECT axial
(A) and coronal MPR (B) images also show markedly
distended loops of small bowel with air-fluid levels. The
abrupt transition point that has resulted in the small bowel
obstruction is marked with arrows.

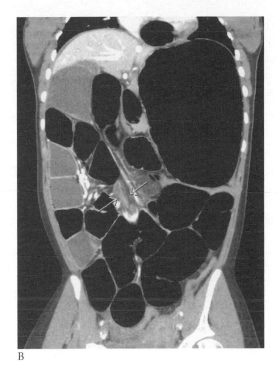

B

FIGURE 2. **Small Bowel Obstruction.** (Continued)

Volvulus

Description: Volvulus is an abnormal twisting (malrotation) of any part of the intestinal tract. The sigmoid and cecum are more commonly affected than the stomach, small intestine, and transverse colon.

Etiology: Most common causes of a volvulus include adhesions, hernias, and tumors.

Epidemiology: A volvulus affecting the small bowel is most commonly seen in children. Colonic volvuluses affect the large bowel. The sigmoid colon is the most common site of involvement accounting for approximately 60% to 75% of all volvulus affecting the colon and is most common in older people. The cecum is the second most common location for colonic volvulus ranging from 25% to 40% of all cases. The transverse colon is the least common site with less than 10% of all volvulus affecting the colon.

Signs and Symptoms: Abdominal pain, abdominal distention, nausea, vomiting, and constipation. Volvulus can result in compromising the blood flow to the affected bowel by strangulation, thus causing necrosis.

Imaging Characteristics:

CT
- Scout film may show the "coffee bean sign" characteristic of a sigmoid volvulus.
- Rotation of the stomach may be seen.
- Bowel dilation and mucosal hyperattenuation may be seen in small bowel ischemia.
- "Whirl sign" or swirling representing the small bowel loop, mesenteric fat, and the superior mesenteric artery and vein.
- Sagittal and coronal MPRs are beneficial in seeing the "whirl sign."
- Useful in identifying the cause of the volvulus.

Treatment: Endoscopic reduction may be used depending on the physical condition of the patient. Laparoscopic surgery may be used to correct the rotation of the bowel. Surgical resection may be needed, especially if there is intestinal necrosis.

Prognosis: Outcome will vary depending on whether the patient has intestinal necrosis. The mortality rate associated with a sigmoid volvulus is 20% to 25%.

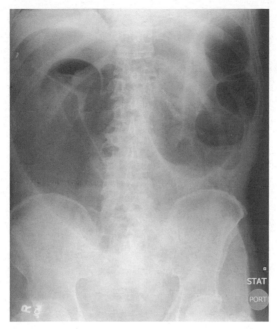

FIGURE 1. **Volvulus.** Plain radiograph of the abdomen showing markedly dilated loops of bowel with a classic "coffee bean" appearance of the dilated sigmoid colon in the right hemiabdomen.

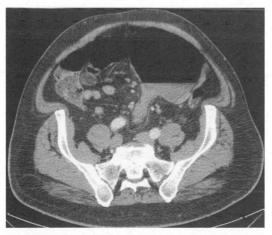

FIGURE 2. **Volvulus.** Axial CECT at the level of the sigmoid volvulus shows the massively dilated sigmoid colon with abrupt narrowing ("bird beaking") at the site of the volvulus.

HEPATOBILIARY

Cavernous Hemangioma

Description: Cavernous hemangiomas are the most common benign hepatic tumors. Found as either single or multiple tumors, they are usually small, measuring 1 to 2 cm in diameter. These tumors are mostly silent with only a small percentage being symptomatic.

Etiology: These vascular malformations are composed of large dilated endothelium-lined vascular channels covered by a fibrous capsule.

Epidemiology: Occur in all age groups. Are more common in females than males. The incidence rate is approximately 1% to 2% in the normal adult population and up to 20% at autopsy.

Signs and Symptoms: Usually in an incidental finding on large symptomatic tumors, upper abdominal pain is experienced.

Imaging Characteristics:

CT
- Noncontrast studies appear hypodense.
- Early peripheral contrast enhancement, whereas the central portion of the lesion remains low density. Sequential scanning over a period of time demonstrates progressive filling of the lesion – central low density progressively becoming smaller.

MRI
- T1-weighted images appear hypointense.
- T2-weighted images appear hyperintense.
- T1-weighted contrast-enhanced images appear hyperintense with increasing signal over 15 to 30 minutes following injection.

Treatment: Surgical intervention is usually not required unless the tumor is large and symptomatic.

Prognosis: Good; these are benign tumors.

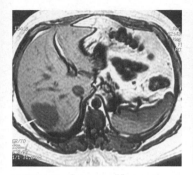

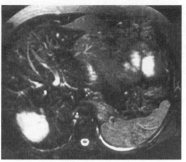

FIGURE 1. Cavernous Hemangioma.
T1-weighted MRI of the liver shows
round low-signal-intensity mass (*arrow*)
in the posterior segment of the right lobe
of the liver.

FIGURE 2. Cavernous Hemangioma.
T2-weighted MRI of the liver shows
this lesion to be very bright (high-signal
intensity).

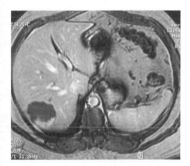

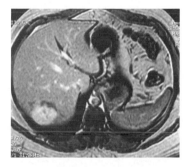

FIGURE 3. Cavernous Hemangioma.
Early postcontrast gradient-echo MRI of
the liver shows peripheral enhancement
of the mass lesion.

FIGURE 4. Cavernous Hemangioma.
Delayed postcontrast gradient-echo MRI
of the liver shows contrast filling of this
lesion.

Choledochal Cysts

Description: A choledochal cyst is a focal dilatation of the bile duct.

Etiology: Choledochal cysts are considered to be a congenital anomaly of the biliary tree.

Epidemiology: More commonly seen in females than males. Patients may be clinically symptomatic before 10 years of age.

Signs and Symptoms: Though not seen in all patients, the classic clinical triad of symptoms includes pain, jaundice, and a palpable abdominal mass in the upper right quadrant.

Imaging Characteristics: A cystic dilatation of the extrahepatic bile, with or without dilatation, of the intrahepatic bile duct.

CT
- Demonstrates a cystic mass in the porta hepatis that appears with an approximate density of water.

MRI
- Low signal from within the cyst is seen on T1-weighted images.
- High signal from within the cyst is seen on T2-weighted images.
- MR cholangiopancreatography (MRCP) is the best noninvasive test for the diagnosis of choledochal cyst.
- MRCP shows localized dilation of the common bile duct.

Treatment: Surgical resection is often performed because of the risk of malignancy associated with this disorder.

Prognosis: If the obstruction is not corrected, infections and chronic liver disease can develop. In the case of a cancerous tumor, complete resection and therapy produce a 5-year survival rate of 30% to 40%.

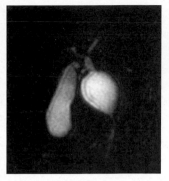

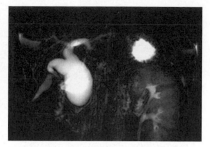

FIGURE 2. **Choledochal Cyst.** Coronal MIP MRCP in a different patient showing a Type IV choledochal cyst.

FIGURE 1. **Choledochal Cyst.** MRCP in the coronal plane shows a fusiform dilatation of the common bile duct. This is consistent with a Type I choledochal cyst.

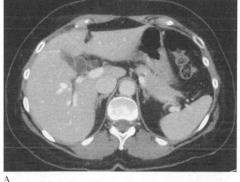

A

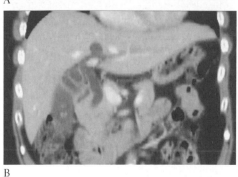

B

FIGURE 3. **Choledochal Cyst.** CECT axial (A) and coronal MPR (B) images show a Type IVa choledochocyst.

Choledocholithiasis

Description: Choledocholithiasis is a calculi or stone in the common bile duct. These calculi usually form in the gallbladder and move into the common bile duct.

Etiology: Stones consisting primarily of cholesterol develop in the gallbladder and enter into the common bile duct.

Epidemiology: Approximately 10% to 15% of patients with cholecystitis have stones in the common bile duct. The incidence rate increases with age and is seen more frequently in females.

Signs and Symptoms: The patient is asymptomatic when there is no obstruction. Abdominal pain in the epigastric region, nausea and vomiting, with a loss of appetite, fever, and jaundice usually indicate an obstruction of the common bile duct. Other signs could include pancreatitis and a palpable gallbladder.

Imaging Characteristics:

CT
- Stones with a high attenuation (hyperdense) may be seen without IV contrast.

MRI
- MR cholangiopancreatography (MRCP) is the best noninvasive study for the diagnoses.
- MRCP demonstrates the stone as hypointense defect in the common bile duct (CBD).

Treatment: Endoscopic retrograde cholangiopancreatography (ERCP) with sphincterotomy and stone removal in most cases. Surgical removal is rarely needed.

Prognosis: Good with early diagnosis and treatment. The patient may experience complications secondary to obstruction of the CBD such as jaundice, cholangitis, and pancreatitis.

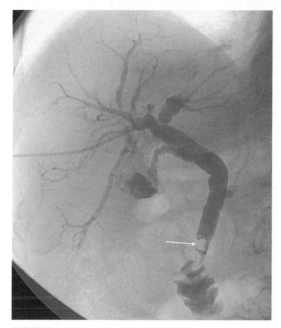

FIGURE 1. Choledocholithiasis. ERCP shows a dilated common bile duct with a distal filling defect (*arrow*) consistent with choledocholithiasis.

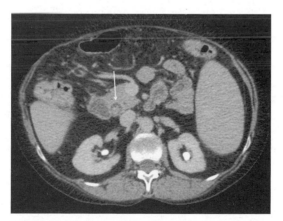

FIGURE 2. Choledocholithiasis. Axial CECT shows a radiodense stone (*arrow*) in the dilated distal common bile duct.

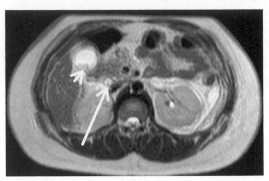

FIGURE 3. **Choledocholithiasis.** MRCP shows multiple hypointense stones in the gallbladder (*short arrow*) as well as a similar-appearing stone in the dilated distal common bile duct (*long arrow*).

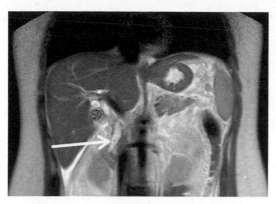

FIGURE 4. **Choledocholithiasis.** Coronal MRCP shows the hypointense stone within the dilated common bile duct (*arrow*).

Fatty Infiltration of the Liver

Description: Fatty infiltration of the liver is the result of excessive depositions of triglycerides and other fats in the liver cells.

Etiology: This condition appears in association with a variety of disorders such as obesity, malnutrition, chemotherapy, alcohol abuse, steroid use, parenteral nutrition, Cushing syndrome, and radiation hepatitis. In the United States, the most common cause is related to alcoholism.

Epidemiology: In the United States, this disorder is commonly associated with the overuse of alcohol.

Signs and Symptoms: Fatty liver is usually "silent" but may be associated with hepatomegaly and abdominal pain in the right upper quadrant.

Imaging Characteristics: CT is the modality of choice for diagnosing fatty infiltration of the liver.

CT
- Fatty infiltrates may be focal or diffusely distributed within the liver.
- Fatty infiltrates demonstrate a lower (hypodense) attenuation in appearance in comparison to the spleen on noncontrast studies.

MRI
- T1- and T2-weighted images may demonstrate an increase in signal when compared to normal liver parenchyma.
- The STIR sequence suppresses the signal from fat when compared to above pulse sequences.

Treatment: Supportive and consists of correcting the underlying condition or eliminating its cause (e.g., alcohol) and focusing on proper nutrition.

Prognosis: Depends on the underlying condition or etiology.

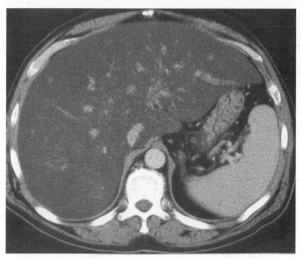

FIGURE 1. **Fatty Infiltration of the Liver.** CT of the abdomen with IV contrast shows mildly enlarged liver. There is diffuse low attenuation of the liver compared to the spleen consistent with fatty infiltration. Note: The contrast opacified hepatic and portal veins against the low-density background of the liver appear bright.

Focal Nodular Hyperplasia

Description: Focal nodular hyperplasia (FNH) is a benign, tumor-like lesion.

Etiology: Though there is no clear cause, a vascular abnormality is suspected.

Epidemiology: It is the second most common benign liver tumor following cavernous hemangioma. May occur in all ages and both sexes; females are predominantly affected between the ages of 30 and 50 years.

Signs and Symptoms: Usually asymptomatic; however, epigastric pain may occur.

Imaging Characteristics:

CT
- Nonenhanced CT shows homogenous hypodense mass.
- IV contrast study shows intense homogeneous enhancement on arterial phase, while the central scar remains hypodense.
- Appears isodense on IV postcontrast study; however, the central scar may show enhancement.

MRI
- T1-weighted images usually appear slightly hypointense.
- T2-weighted images usually appear slightly hyperintense.
- May appear isointense on T1- and T2-weighted images with surrounding liver tissue.
- T1-weighted IV postgadolinium images appear slightly hyperintense immediately following contrast.
- Delayed T1-weighted IV postgadolinium images appear slightly hyperintense with a partially enhanced central scar.

Treatment: No treatment is required.

Prognosis: Good; this is a benign incidental finding.

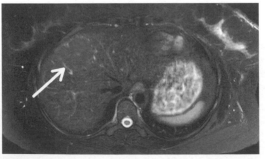

FIGURE 1. **Focal Nodular Hyperplasia.** Axial T2W turbo spin echo (TSE) shows a mildly lobulated mass in the liver (*arrow*) with a hyperintense central scar and radiating septa.

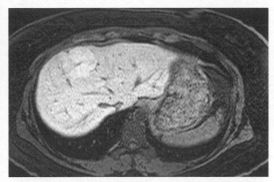

FIGURE 2. **Focal Nodular Hyperplasia.** Arterial phase postcontrast T1W fat saturation sequence shows homogeneous enhancement with a hypointense central scar.

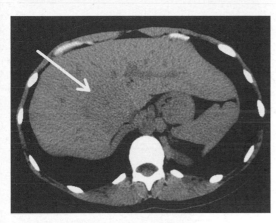

FIGURE 3. **Focal Nodular Hyperplasia.** Axial NECT shows a low-attenuation mass in the liver (*arrow*) with a hypodense central scar.

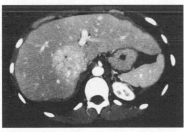

A

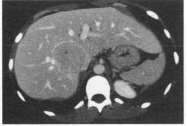

B

FIGURE 4. **Focal Nodular Hyperplasia.** Axial CECT images in the hepatic arterial phase (A) and portal venous phase (B) show early transient enhancement with an unenhanced central scar.

Hemochromatosis

Description: Hemochromatosis is a hereditary disorder in which the small bowel absorbs an excessive amount of iron.

Etiology: Results from an excessive absorption of iron. The iron is initially stored in the hepatocytes as the disease progresses and then spreads into other organs such as the pancreas, GI tract, kidneys, heart, joints, and endocrine glands such as the pituitary gland, resulting in the destruction of these tissues.

Epidemiology: Hemochromatosis usually manifests in the fourth and fifth decades of life. Males are more affected than females.

Signs and Symptoms: Fatigue, impotence, arthralgia, and hepatomegaly are common in early stages. Later stages may include skin bronzing, diabetes mellitus, cirrhosis, and hepatocellular carcinoma.

Imaging Characteristics: Increased liver attenuation by deposition of iron. Normal liver attenuation is 40 to 70 HU.

CT
- Detected with noncontrast-enhanced examination of the abdomen.
- 70 HU or greater is an indication of iron overload.

MRI
- More sensitive than noncontrast-enhanced CT.
- Affected hepatocytes appear with decreased signal as a result of paramagnetic effect of the ferric iron Fe^{3+}, thus shortening T1 and T2 relaxation times of nearby protons.
- Best seen on gradient-echo T2-weighted images which show magnetic inhomogeneities better than spin-echo images.

Treatment: Is directed at removing the iron (phlebotomy) before it can produce serious irreversible liver damage. Iron supplements are restricted.

Prognosis: Normal life can be expected if iron reduction is initiated prior to the development of liver damage (cirrhosis).

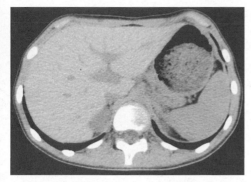

FIGURE 1.
Hemochromatosis. Axial NECT shows a relatively hyperdense liver compared to the spleen and hepatic vessels in a patient with primary hemochromatosis.

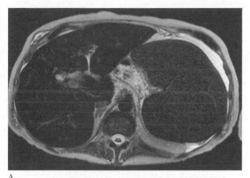

A

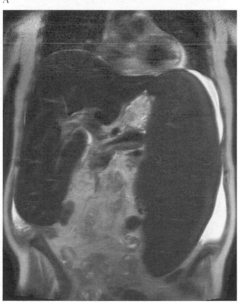

B

FIGURE 2.
Hemochromatosis. Axial (A) and coronal (B) T2W images show marked signal loss in the liver and spleen with significant hepatosplenomegaly in a patient with secondary hemochromatosis.

Hepatic Adenoma

Description: Hepatic adenomas are benign tumors.

Etiology: Tends to occur in young females with a history of oral contraceptives. Males who take anabolic steroids may be at risk.

Epidemiology: Approximately 90% occur in young females.

Signs and Symptoms: Small hepatic adenomas are usually asymptomatic. Patients may present with acute abdominal pain, related to hemorrhaging into the tumor.

Imaging Characteristics: Hepatic adenoma typically measures 8 to 15 cm on average, and may present as a mass in the upper right quadrant or as hepatomegaly. The presence of fat or hemorrhage within the mass is suggestive of a hepatic adenoma.

CT
- Nonenhanced study shows tumor as isodense to normal liver parenchyma.
- IV contrast shows homogenous enhancement in arterial phase, similar to hepatocellular carcinoma, metastatic disease, and focal nodular hyperplasia.
- Appears isodense to liver parenchyma on delayed IV contrast images.
- Difficult to differentiate between focal nodular hyperplasia, hepatocellular carcinoma, and metastatic disease.
- There is no central scar as seen in focal nodular hyperplasia.

MRI
- More sensitive in detecting fat and hemorrhage.
- T1-weighted images show the tumor as isointense to slightly hypointense to the liver parenchyma.
- T2-weighted images show the tumor as isointense to hypointense signal.
- Postgadolinium images show the tumor as hyperintense.
- MR elastography (MRE) demonstrates that benign tumors have a lesser mean shear stiffness than malignant tumors.

Treatment: Surgery is usually advised to remove risk of hemorrhage, though hepatic adenoma may develop into hepatocellular carcinoma (HCC).

Prognosis: Good; this is a benign tumor. There is, however, a risk of hemorrhage associated with this tumor.

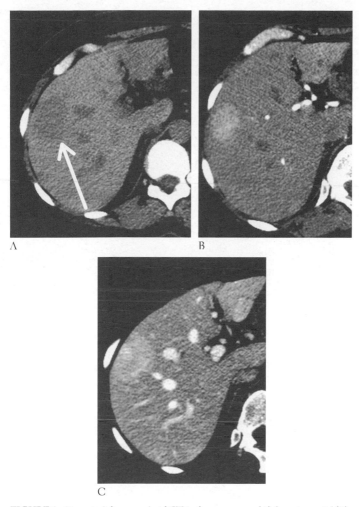

FIGURE 1. Hepatic Adenoma. Axial CT in the precontrast (A), hepatic arterial (B), and portal venous (C) phases show a hypodense subcapsular mass in the right lobe of the liver that enhances homogeneously. There is no central scar.

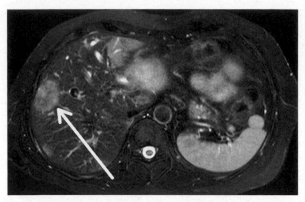

FIGURE 2. **Hepatic Adenoma.** T2W axial MR image shows the mass to be hyperintense to the surrounding liver.

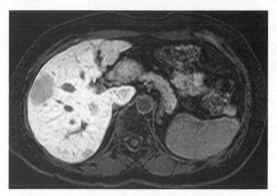

FIGURE 3. Hepatic Adenoma. After administration of Eovist, the mass remains hypointense to the surrounding liver consistent with an adenoma.

Hepatic Cysts

Description: Simple hepatic cysts found in the liver.

Etiology: Liver cysts are thought to be congenital.

Epidemiology: These lesions are commonly found in roughly 5% to 10% of the general population.

Signs and Symptoms: Hepatic cysts are asymptomatic. They are usually an incidental finding.

Imaging Characteristics: Hepatic cysts may appear as single or multiple cysts.

CT
- Appear as a homogeneous, well-defined, round or oval-shaped, and thin-walled lesion.
- The cysts have a near-water attenuation value that should not enhance with IV contrast.

MRI
- T1-weighted images appear hypointense.
- T2-weighted images appear hyperintense.
- T1-weighted contrast-enhanced images will show no enhancement.

Treatment: There is no treatment required for hepatic cysts.

Prognosis: Since these lesions are incidental findings and are asymptomatic with no known side effects, the prognosis for these cysts is good.

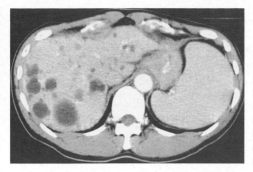

FIGURE 1. **Liver Cysts.**
CT of the abdomen with
IV contrast demonstrates
multiple low-density lesions
in the liver. These lesions
have a near-water CT
attenuation value and smooth
margins consistent with cysts.

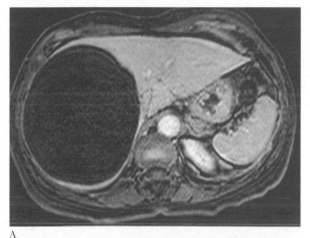

A

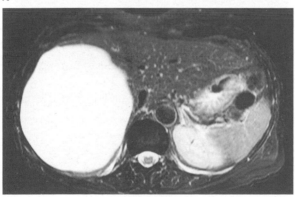

B

FIGURE 2. **Hepatic Cysts.** Axial T1W (A) and T2W (B) images
show the cyst follows the signal characteristics of water.

Hepatic Metastases

Description: Metastatic spread of cancer to the liver involves the deposit of cancer cells into the liver parenchyma. Metastatic liver disease occurs more frequently than primary liver malignancies.

Etiology: Liver metastases can originate from essentially any primary malignancy, but most commonly spread from the gastrointestinal tract, especially, the colon. Other cancers that frequently metastasize to the liver include gastric, pancreatic, breast, lung, ovary, kidney, and carcinoid tumors of the intestinal tract which tend to occur in the terminal ileum or appendix.

Epidemiology: The liver is the second most common site (lungs are the most commonly affected) for metastatic spread of cancer.

Signs and Symptoms: May present with abdominal pain, jaundice, and possibly a palpable mass.

Imaging Characteristics: Contrast-enhanced CT is the modality of choice. MRI is useful when CT is inconclusive.

CT
◆ Well-defined low-attenuation (hypodense) solid masses when compared to the liver parenchyma on noncontrast studies.
◆ Some tumors may show contrast enhancement.
◆ Calcifications or hemorrhage may be seen in the metastatic masses on noncontrast CT.

MRI
◆ T1-weighted images show hypointense metastatic lesion.
◆ T2-weighted images may show hypointense, isointense, or hyperintense metastatic lesions.
◆ Gadolinium-enhanced T1-weighted images show hypointense lesions.

Treatment: Depends on the cancer staging. Chemotherapy may be used singularly or in combination with conservative surgical resection when metastasis is localized to three or fewer segments.

Prognosis: Poor; depends on the stage of the primary cancer.

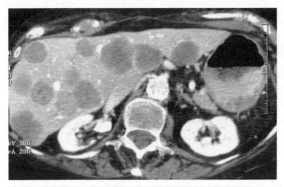

FIGURE 1. **Liver Metastasis.** Contrast-enhanced CT of the abdomen demonstrates multiple round hypodense lesions throughout the liver, consistent with liver metastasis.

Hepatoma

Description: A hepatoma, also known as hepatocellular carcinoma (HCC), is the most common primary malignant liver tumor. It accounts for approximately 75% of liver cancers.

Etiology: Risk factors associated with hepatoma include hepatitis B infection, alcohol-induced cirrhosis, aflatoxin (a mold that grows on rice and peanuts)-contaminated food, anabolic steroids, Thorotrast (thorium dioxide, a contrast medium formerly used in liver radiography), and immunosuppressive agents.

Epidemiology: In the United States, incidence rates range from one to five new cases per 100,000 population per year. The average age of detection is between the fifth and sixth decades of life. Males are affected more than females at a ratio of 3:1. The incidence rate among individuals from China, Southeast Asia, western and southern Africa, Taiwan, and Hong Kong is high.

Signs and Symptoms: Patient may present with a palpable mass, abdominal pain in the right upper quadrant (RUQ), hepatomegaly, weight loss, and nausea and vomiting, and may be a known cirrhosis patient.

Imaging Characteristics:

CT
- Appears hypodense on noncontrast study.
- CT with IV contrast show variable enhancement.

MRI
- T1-weighted images appear hypointense.
- T2-weighted images appear hyperintense.
- T1-weighted contrast-enhanced images show variable enhancement.

Treatment: Surgical intervention to remove the tumor prolongs life and may improve the patient's quality of life. The presence of cirrhosis reduces the patient's prognosis. Radiation therapy and chemotherapy are used to provide some degree of palliation.

Prognosis: Surgical resection of the tumor is the treatment of choice. Unfortunately, 85% to 90% of the cases are not surgical resectable.

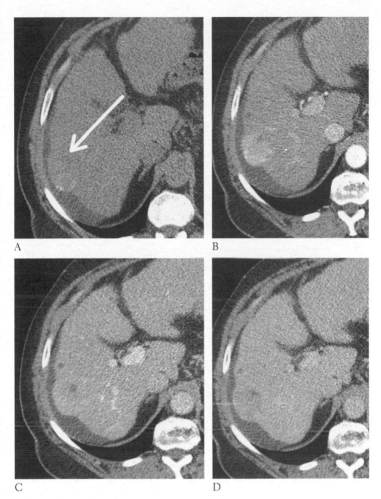

FIGURE 1. **Hepatoma.** Noncontrast (A), hepatic arterial (B), portal venous (C), and delayed (D) phases axial CT images show a low-attenuation mass with calcification in the right lobe of the liver that becomes hyperdense and then washes out becoming hypodense to the surrounding liver.

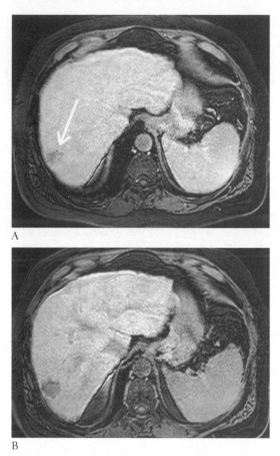

A

B

FIGURE 2. **Hepatoma.** Postcontrast T1W (A) image and
delayed T1W (B) image show similar findings to the CT.

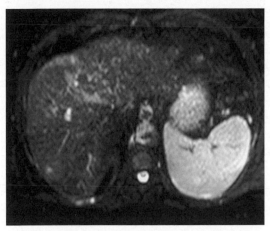

FIGURE 3. **Hepatoma.** T2W image shows the hepatoma to be slightly hyperintense to the surrounding liver with a central area of hyperintensity due to necrosis.

PANCREAS

Pancreatic Adenocarcinoma

Description: Pancreatic adenocarcinoma is the second most common visceral malignancy and the fifth leading cause of cancer mortality.

Etiology: Though there is no known cause, there is evidence that suggests a link to inhalation or absorption of certain carcinogens found in cigarettes, foods high in fat and protein, food additives, industrial chemicals (betanaphthalene, benzidine, and urea). Additional possible predisposing factors are chronic pancreatitis, diabetes mellitus, and chronic alcohol abuse.

Epidemiology: There are approximately 28,000 new cases diagnosed annually with about 26,000 deaths. It occurs most commonly between the fourth and seventh decades of life. The majority of these tumors are located in the head of the pancreas.

Signs and Symptoms: Patients usually present with weight loss, abdominal pain, and jaundice. Jaundice is caused by an obstruction of the bile ducts by the pancreatic tumor (head).

Imaging Characteristics: Contrast CT is the preferred imaging modality. MRI is used in difficult cases.

CT and MRI
- Mass in the head of the pancreas (majority 66%).
- Dilated bile ducts, pancreatic duct secondary to obstruction of the distal common bile duct (CBD) by the tumor in the head of the pancreas.
- Invasion or encasement of adjacent vascular structures by pancreatic tumor.
- Liver metastasis.
- Enlarged metastatic lymph nodes.

Treatment: Though surgery offers the best hope for cure, roughly 80% of the patients at diagnosis are ineligible for curative treatment. Radiation therapy may be helpful. Chemotherapy has not proven to improve the patient's condition.

Prognosis: Poor. The average survival following pancreatic resection is approximately 17 months.

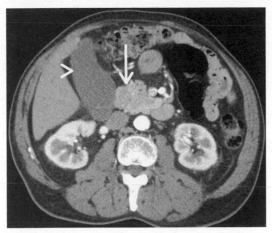

FIGURE 1. **Pancreatic Adenocarcinoma.** CECT shows
a low-attenuation mass in the head of the pancreas (*arrow*)
which is constricting the common bile duct evidenced by the
distended gallbladder (*arrowhead*).

Pancreatic Pseudocyst

Description: Pancreatic pseudocysts are composed of a collection of cellular debris, old blood, and pancreatic fluid that has become encapsulated in a fibrous sac.

Etiology: Pseudocysts of the pancreas may occur as a result of pancreatic inflammation and trauma.

Epidemiology: Patients who have recently experienced a bout of acute pancreatitis or trauma to the pancreas are potential candidates to develop pseudocysts.

Signs and Symptoms: Patients present with a palpable mass, abdominal pain, nausea and vomiting, loss of appetite, and jaundice.

Imaging Characteristics:

CT
- Appears as a well-defined, round, low-density, thick- or thin-walled capsule and has a near-water attenuation value.

MRI
- The pseudocyst will appear with a low-signal (hypointense) region on T1-weighted images and with a high signal on T2-weighted images.

Treatment: Pancreatic pseudocysts may resolve spontaneously. For those that do not resolve or increase in size, drainage is usually required either through a CT-guided catheter or surgical drainage.

Prognosis: Depends on complications associated with extent and severity of the pseudocyst and treatment. In the more serious cases, there can be a high morbidity and mortality rate.

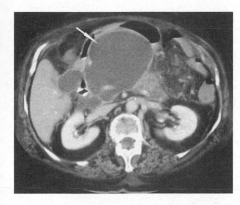

FIGURE 1. Pancreatic Pseudocyst. CT of the abdomen with IV contrast demonstrates a large, round, low-density mass (*arrow*) in the region of the head of the pancreas with displacement of the stomach and duodenum. This cystic mass has a near-water CT attenuation value consistent with a cyst.

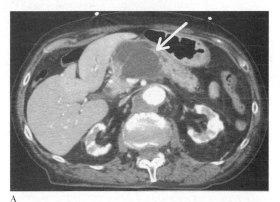

A

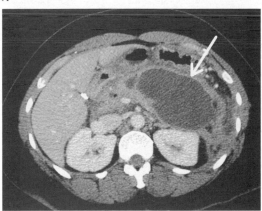

B

FIGURE 2. Pancreatic Pseudocyst. Axial CECT images show a large fluid attenuation, unenhancing cyst in the body (A) and tail (B) of the pancreas. These are consistent with a pseudocyst.

Pancreatitis

Description: Pancreatitis is an inflammation of the pancreas, and occurs in acute and chronic forms. The difference between the acute and chronic forms is based on the restoration of normal pancreatic function in the former and permanent residual damage in the latter.

Etiology: The most common cause of pancreatitis is alcoholism. Other causes include gallstones, trauma, pancreatic cancer, certain drugs, post endoscopic retrograde cholangiopancreatography (ERCP), and metabolic disorders (hypertriglyceridemia, hypercalcemia, renal failure).

Epidemiology: The incidence rate is between 10 and 20 per 100,000 population. Acute pancreatitis can occur at any time; however, chronic pancreatitis tends to occur between 35 and 45 years of age and is usually linked with alcohol intake. Males and females are equally affected.

Signs and Symptoms: Patients may present with abdominal pain, nausea and vomiting, mild abdominal distention, fever, hypotension, mild jaundice, reduced or absent bowel sounds, umbilical discoloration (Cullen sign), and pleural effusion.

Imaging Characteristics: CT is the imaging modality of choice.

CT
- Diffuse enlargement of the pancreas.
- Soft-tissue stranding of the peripancreatic fat and thickening of the fascia.
- Intrapancreatic and peripancreatic fluid collection.
- Pancreatic pseudocyst may be seen.
- Pancreatic calcification may be seen in chronic pancreatitis.

Treatment: Medical treatment is mostly symptomatic with the focus being to prevent and treat the complications. Pancreatic abscess and pseudocysts can be treated with CT-guided catheter drainage. Surgery may be necessary in some cases.

Prognosis: Depends on the underlying condition or etiology as well as the complications associated with pancreatitis.

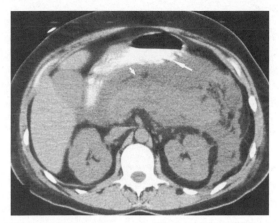

FIGURE 1. Severe Pancreatitis. CT of the abdomen without IV contrast demonstrates diffuse enlargement of the pancreas. Fluid collection noted along the anterior aspect of the pancreas within the lesser sac (*short arrow*) with displacement of the barium opacified stomach anteriorly (*long arrow*). Note: There is thickening of the renal fascia on the left kidney.

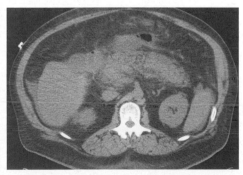

FIGURE 2. Pancreatitis. Axial NECT shows findings consistent with acute pancreatitis including an enlarged edematous pancreas with marked peripancreatic stranding and ascites.

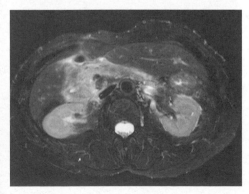

FIGURE 3. Pancreatitis. Axial T2W MR shows an enlarged hyperintense pancreas due to pancreatic edema with associated hyperintense fat stranding.

GENITOURINARY

Agenesis of the Kidney

Description: Renal agenesis is the congenital absence of one of the kidneys.

Etiology: Renal agenesis is a congenital anomaly.

Epidemiology: Unilateral agenesis of the kidney occurs in approximately 1 out of every 500 patients, and is more commonly found in males than females with a 3:1 ratio.

Signs and Symptoms: In many cases renal agenesis is an incidental finding.

Imaging Characteristics:

CT and MRI
- Absence of a kidney.
- Compensatory hypertrophy of existing kidney, renal vein, and adrenal gland.

Treatment: There is no treatment for this condition. Patient education and monitoring for preventative measures might be advised.

Prognosis: Depending on renal function, the patient may live a normal life.

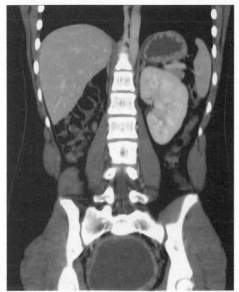

A

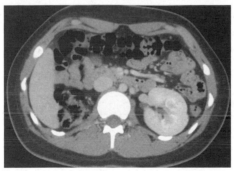

B

FIGURE 1. **Agenesis of the Kidney.** Coronal MPR (A) and axial (B) CECT images show a congenitally absent right kidney with displacement of the bowel into the renal fossa on the right and compensatory enlargement of the left kidney.

Angiomyolipoma

Description: Angiomyolipomas are fairly common benign renal tumors composed of three components: (1) fat, (2) blood vessels, and (3) smooth muscles. The term *hamartoma* is associated with a benign mass composed of disorganized tissues normally found in an organ, while the term *choristoma* implies a benign mass of disorganized tissues not normally found in an organ.

Etiology: A tumor composed of an overgrowth of mature cells and tissues normally present in the affected area (i.e., blood vessels, smooth muscle tissue, and fat).

Epidemiology: Angiomyolipomas are more commonly seen in females than males ranging from 40 to 60 years of age. About 20% of all patients diagnosed with angiomyolipomas have multiple, bilateral masses, and are associated with tuberous sclerosis.

Signs and Symptoms: Patients present with abdominal pain, palpable mass, hemorrhage, and hematuria.

Imaging Characteristics:

CT
- The detection of the fat in this renal mass assist with confirming the diagnosis of angiomyolipoma.

MRI
- T1- and T2-weighted images will appear with high signal (hyperintense).
- T1-weighted fat-suppression technique allows fat within the tumor to be distinguished from hemorrhage.

Treatment: Surgical intervention is required if life-threatening hemorrhaging occurs. Angioembolization can also be used.

Prognosis: Angiomyolipoma are benign tumors. Mortality is usually secondary to bleeding or hemorrhage of the tumor.

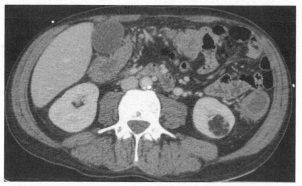

FIGURE 1. Angiomyolipoma. CECT shows a well-demarcated fat containing mass in the left kidney with minimal enhancement.

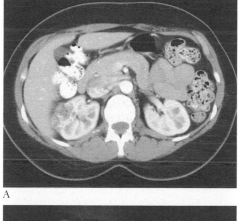

A

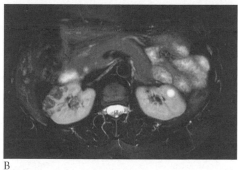

B

FIGURE 2. Angiomyolipoma. CECT (A) shows a mass arising from the right renal cortex which appears to contain fat. This is confirmed on a fat-suppressed T2W image (B) which demonstrates signal loss in the mass.

Horseshoe Kidney

Description: A horseshoe kidney is a congenital anomaly characterized by the fusion of the lower (90%) or upper (10%) poles of the kidney. This produces a horseshoe-shaped structure continuous across the midline and anterior to the great vessels.

Etiology: Horseshoe kidney is a congenital anomaly.

Epidemiology: This anomaly is considered to be common and is found in about 1 in every 500 patients.

Signs and Symptoms: This condition is usually asymptomatic but there can be complications such as ureteropelvic junction (UPJ) obstruction, infections, and stone formation.

Imaging Characteristics:

CT
- Demonstrates a horseshoe-shaped kidney fused more commonly at the lower pole (90%) or at the upper pole (10%) of the time.

MRI
- T1-weighted imaging is best used to visualize this anatomical renal anomaly.

Treatment: This congenital anomaly is usually seen as an incidental finding and requires no treatment.

Prognosis: Depending on renal function, the patient should live a normal life.

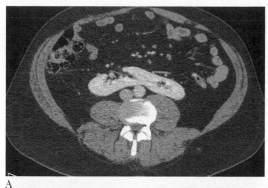

A

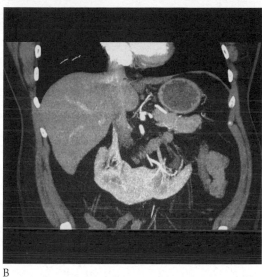

B

FIGURE 1. **Horseshoe Kidney.** Axial (A) and coronal MPR
(B) CECT shows fusion of the kidneys across the midline.

Perinephric Hematoma

Description: A perinephric hematoma is a collection of blood that is confined to Gerota fascia (i.e., perirenal fascia) and arises as a result of blunt or penetrating trauma to the kidney.

Etiology: Blunt or penetrating trauma to the abdominal area.

Epidemiology: Renal injuries occur in approximately 10% of trauma victims. Most renal injuries are associated with motor vehicle accidents. It is common for a hemorrhage to occur in the perinephrotic space following a renal biopsy.

Signs and Symptoms: Depending on the extent of the injury and time to treatment, patients may present with abdominal pain, an open wound, signs of internal bleeding with blood in the urine, increased heart rate, declining blood pressure, and hypovolemic shock, nausea and vomiting, decreased alertness, and moist clammy skin.

Imaging Characteristics: Contrast-enhanced CT is the modality of choice for the evaluation of abdominal or renal trauma.

CT
- Hyperdense in appearance on acute noncontrast studies.
- Hypodense area surrounding the contrast-enhanced kidney.
- Shows associated laceration of kidney.
- Follow-up CT for stable patient with conservative treatment to monitor resolution of hematoma.

Treatment: Surgical intervention may be required in emergent situations for the hemodynamically unstable patient. Conservative treatment for the stable patient may include bed rest, analgesics, and patient monitoring.

Prognosis: Depends on the extent of the injury, patient response to treatment, and any other associated injuries.

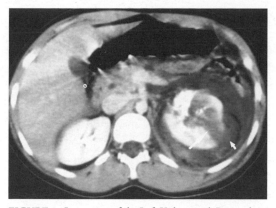

FIGURE 1. Laceration of the Left Kidney with Perinephric Hematoma. CT of the abdomen with IV contrast shows low-density areas of the parenchyma of the left kidney consistent with deep (*long arrow*) Grade 3 laceration and hematoma. There is also a hematoma (*short arrow*) surrounding the left kidney.

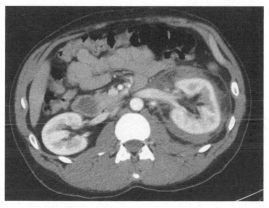

FIGURE 2. Perinephric Hematoma. Axial CECT shows fluid density around the left kidney consistent with a perinephric hematoma.

Polycystic Kidney Disease

Description: Adult polycystic kidney disease (PKD) is an inherited disorder, characterized by multiple fluid-filled cysts of varying sizes. These cysts cause lobulated enlargements of the kidneys that result in cystic compression and progressive failure of the renal tissue.

Etiology: Adult polycystic kidney disease is a hereditary (autosomal dominant) disorder.

Epidemiology: Incidence rate is between 1 and 5 in 1000. Males and females are equally affected. Usually diagnosed between the third and fourth decades of life. PKD accounts for 5% to 10% of patients with end-stage renal disease.

Signs and Symptoms: Patients may present with hypertension, hematuria, palpable kidneys, hepatomegaly, abdominal pain, and flank pain. An association with PKD and the presence of cerebral berry aneurysms exist.

Imaging Characteristics:

CT
- Multiple hypodense or cystic masses involving one or both kidneys.
- Enlarged kidneys.

MRI
- Enlarged kidneys with multiple cysts that have a low signal on T1-weighted images and a high signal on T2-weighted images.

Treatment: PKD is incurable. Treatment is aimed at preserving renal parenchyma and preventing infectious complications. Managing hypertension helps prevent rapid deterioration in function. Progressive renal failure requires treatment such as dialysis or, rarely, kidney transplant.

Prognosis: Slowly progressive, with a variable outcome. End-stage renal disease occurs in 70% of patients by age 65.

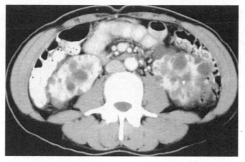

FIGURE 1. **Adult Polycystic Kidney Disease.** CT of the abdomen with IV contrast demonstrates enlarged bilateral kidneys with numerous cysts of varying sizes.

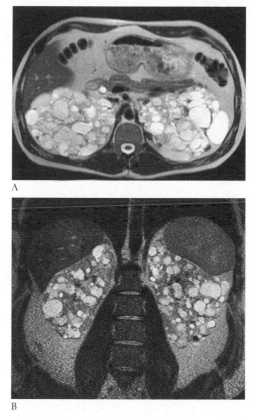

A

B

FIGURE 2. **Polycystic Kidney Disease.** Axial (A) and coronal (B) T2W images show enlarged kidneys which are nearly replaced with cysts. These cysts have high signal characteristics similar to fluid.

Pyelonephritis

Description: Pyelonephritis is an inflammation of the kidney and renal pelvis.

Etiology: Bacterial infection usually involving *E. coli* in 70% to 80% of cases.

Epidemiology: Occurs more commonly in females than males.

Signs and Symptoms: Urinary tract infections (UTI) typically present in the patient with chills, fever, lower back pain on the affected side, and nausea and vomiting.

Imaging Characteristics: CT with IV contrast is the modality of choice when imaging patients with acute bacterial pyelonephritis. CT with IV contrast acquired during the corticomedullary phase (30 seconds following injection) and during either the nephrographic phase (70 to 90 seconds following injection) or the excretory phase (5 minutes following the injection).

CT
- Enlarged kidney.
- Perinephric stranding.
- Hydronephrosis.
- Abnormalities seen on IV postcontrast as wedge-shaped zones of decreased attenuation.

MRI
- Enlarged kidney.
- Perinephric stranding.
- Hydronephrosis.
- Perinephric fluid best seen on IV postcontrast images.
- T1-weighted fat-suppression images may show proteinaceous material in the renal tubules as high-signal substance.

Treatment: All symptoms usually resolve within 72 hours following administration of the appropriate antibiotic therapy.

Prognosis: Most patients experience full recovery.

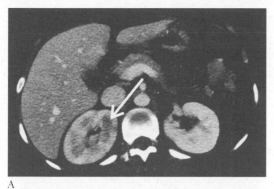

FIGURE 1. **Pyelonephritis.** Axial (Λ) and coronal (B) CECTs show multiple wedge-shaped areas of decreased attenuation predominately in the right kidney.

Renal Artery Stenosis

Description: The most common cause of correctable hypertension is stenosis of the renal artery. Hypertension of the renal artery can occur as a result of either atherosclerosis or fibromuscular dysplasia.

Etiology: Results from the accumulation of atherosclerotic plaques or fibromuscular dysplasia in the renal artery.

Epidemiology: Hypertension from renal artery stenosis occurs in less than 5% of all patients with hypertension. Atherosclerosis occurs mainly in older people. Fibromuscular dysplasia is more commonly seen in young females than young males.

Signs and Symptoms: Patients present with hypertension.

Imaging Characteristics: Noninvasive studies include captopril renal nuclear medicine scan and magnetic resonance angiography (MRA) with gadolinium. Conventional angiography is the gold standard, but it is invasive.

MRI and CT
◆ Atherosclerotic narrowing involves the proximal renal artery close to its origin.
◆ Fibromuscular dysplasia causes a beading (string of pearls) appearance and involves the distal two-thirds of the renal artery as well as other peripheral branches.

Treatment: Methods of treatment include angioplasty, stenting, and surgical revascularization.

Prognosis: Good with early diagnosis and treatment.

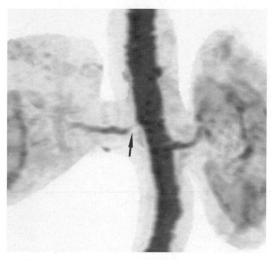

FIGURE 1. Renal Artery Stenosis. MR angiogram of the abdominal aorta shows severe narrowing (*arrow*) of the proximal right renal artery close to its origin from the aorta. Left renal artery is normal.

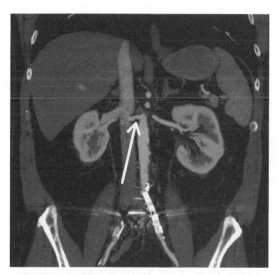

FIGURE 2. Renal Artery Stenosis. Coronal MIP CT angiogram shows atheromatous plaque along the aortic wall and small filling defect (*arrow*) in the proximal right renal artery resulting in renal artery stenosis.

Renal Calculus

Description: Renal calculi (kidney stones) may form anywhere throughout the urinary tract. They usually develop in the renal pelvis or the calyces of the kidneys. The majority of renal stones are composed of calcium salts. Kidney stones vary in size and may be solitary or multiple. They may remain in the renal pelvis or enter the ureter.

Etiology: The exact cause is unknown; however, predisposing factors include dehydration (increased concentration of calculus-forming substances), infection (changes in pH), obstruction (urinary stasis, such as may be seen in spinal cord injuries), metabolic disorders (e.g., hyperparathyroidism, renal tubular acidosis, elevated uric acid [usually without gout]), defective metabolism of oxalate, genetic defect in metabolism of cystine, and excessive intake of vitamin D or dietary calcium.

Epidemiology: Renal calculi result in roughly 1 per 1000 hospitalizations annually. They typically occur between 30 and 50 years of age. Most occur in the third decade of life. Calcium stones affect males more than females by a ratio of 3:1.

Signs and Symptoms: Patients may present with back pain (renal colic), pain radiating into groin area, hematuria, dysuria, polyuria, chills, and fever associated with infection due to obstruction, nausea, vomiting, diarrhea, abdominal distention, and costovertebral angle tenderness.

Imaging Characteristics: Noncontrast CT of the abdomen and pelvis is the imaging modality of choice and is gradually replacing the IVP.

CT

- Noncontrast CT demonstrates calcified stone in the kidney or ureter.
- May show hydronephrosis and hydroureter.
- May show perinephric soft-tissue stranding.

Treatment: Treatment includes pain management, fluid management, straining urine for urine analysis and stone collection, and extracorporeal shock wave lithotripsy. Surgery is rarely indicated.

Prognosis: A good prognosis is expected with complete return to the patient's previous state of health.

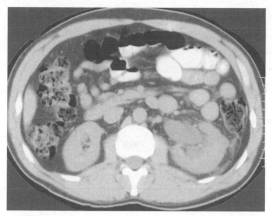

FIGURE 1. **Kidney Hydronephrosis.** CT of the abdomen without IV contrast demonstrates mild left hydronephrosis. There is left perinephric soft-tissue stranding.

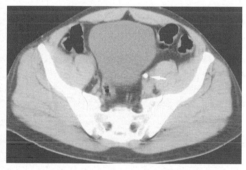

FIGURE 2. **Kidney Calculus.** CT of the pelvis on the same patient above (see Figure 1) demonstrating a calcified stone (*arrow*) of the left distal ureter.

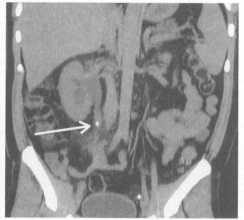

FIGURE 3. **Renal Calculus.** Coronal NECT shows a dense stone in the right ureter with secondary hydronephrosis due to obstruction.

Renal Cell Carcinoma

Description: Renal cell carcinoma (RCC) is the most common malignancy affecting the kidney.

Etiology: The cause of renal cell carcinoma is unknown; however, it is known to arise from the proximal convoluted tubule.

Epidemiology: Approximately 30,000 new cases are diagnosed annually with about 12,000 deaths. Males are affected more than females at a ratio of 2:1. The average age of occurrence appears between the fifth and sixth decades of life.

Signs and Symptoms: Patients may present with a solid renal mass (6 to 7 cm), hematuria, abdominal mass, anemia, flank pain, hypertension, and weight loss.

Imaging Characteristics:

CT
- Precontrast studies show hypodense or isodense renal mass.
- Post IV contrast study shows enhancing mass.

MRI
- T1-weighted images appear isointense.
- T2-weighted images appear hyperintense to parenchyma.
- Postcontrast T1-weighted images appear hyperintense with heterogeneous enhancement.

Treatment: Surgical removal of the kidney (nephrectomy) when the cancer is confined to only one kidney. Radiation and chemotherapy are of little value in treating RCC.

Prognosis: Depends on the staging at the time of diagnosis.

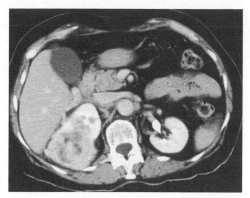

FIGURE 1. **Renal Cell Carcinoma.** CT of the abdomen with IV contrast demonstrates a large solid round mass of the posterior aspect of the right kidney. Note: There are low-density areas within the mass consistent with necrosis. There is also some contrast enhancement.

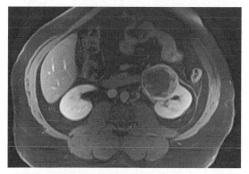

FIGURE 2. **Renal Cell Carcinoma.** Postcontrast axial T1W image shows enhancement of the solid portions of the left renal mass.

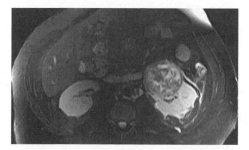

FIGURE 3. **Renal Cell Carcinoma.** T2W image shows areas of increased signal in the mass consistent with central necrosis of the renal cell carcinoma.

Renal Infarct

Description: A renal infarct is a localized area of necrosis in the kidney.

Etiology: An acute infarct of the kidney may follow a thromboembolic (most common), renal artery occlusion (due to atherosclerosis), blunt abdominal trauma, or a sudden, complete renal venous occlusion.

Epidemiology: The most common cause of renal emboli occurs in patients with atrial arrhythmias or patients who have a history of a myocardial infarction. In addition, patients who have experienced blunt abdominal trauma may develop renal emboli.

Signs and Symptoms: This condition may go unnoticed; however, some patients may experience pain with tenderness in the region of the costo-vertebral angle of the affected side.

Imaging Characteristics: Contrast-enhanced CT is the preferred modality. Convention renal arteriogram is the gold standard for the evaluation of an occlusion of renal artery or its branches.

CT
- Contrast-enhanced images show a wedge-shaped hypodense area as the affected region.

MRI
- T1-weighted and T2-weighted images may demonstrate a lower than normal signal in the affected area.
- T1-weighted postcontrast images demonstrate a wedge-shaped low-signal area of the renal parenchyma.
- MRA may show occlusion of the main renal artery or its branches.

Treatment: Thrombectomy or embolectomy may be useful in the early stage.

Prognosis: Depends on early detection and treatment.

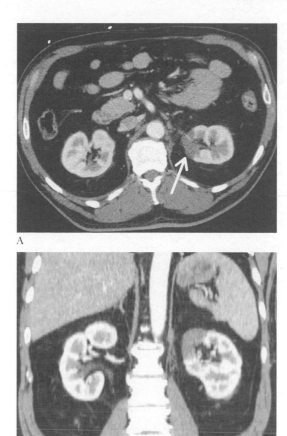

A

B

FIGURE 1. **Renal Infarct.** Axial (A) and coronal MPR
(B) CECTs show a wedge-shaped area of nonenhancing
renal cortex in the upper pole of the left kidney as a result of
infarction.

Wilm Tumor

Description: The most common type of renal cancer in children and the fifth most common cancer affecting children is a Wilm tumor. Wilm tumor may also be called nephroblastoma (a malignant tumor arising from the embryonic kidney).

Etiology: The majority of cases are sporadic. Only about 5% are inherited.

Epidemiology: About 87% of all renal neoplasms are Wilm tumor. About 80% of this tumor presents between 1 and 5 years of age, with the peak age at the time of diagnosis between 3 and 4 years old. The incidence rate of Wilm tumor is about 1 per 100,000 population. Bilateral involvement may be seen in 10% of cases.

Signs and Symptoms: The most common sign is an abdominal mass. Abdominal pain may be present in 30% to 40% of the cases. Hypertension, hematuria, and anemia are other signs and symptoms associated with Wilm tumor.

Imaging Characteristics: Ultrasound initial modality of choice, especially for pediatric patients and radiation dose.

CT
- Appears as a large, spherical, intrarenal mass with a well-defined rim.
- Calcification may be seen in 5% to 10% of noncontrast cases.
- Helpful in staging and metastatic spread (lung metastases are more frequently involved than the liver).

MRI
- Appears with hypointense signal on T1-weighted images.
- Hyperintense signal on T2-weighted images.
- Wilm tumor usually appears inhomogeneous on postgadolinium examinations.

Treatment: Surgery with postchemotherapy with unilateral involvement. Surgery is not an option for bilateral disease.

Prognosis: With appropriate therapy and early detection, a good outcome is expected.

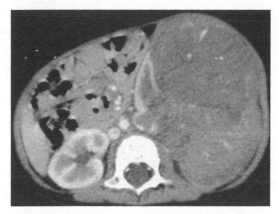

FIGURE 1. **Wilm Tumor.** Axial CECT shows a large heterogenous mass arising from the left kidney and filling the entire left hemiabdomen.

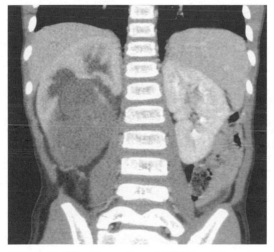

FIGURE 2. **Wilm Tumor.** Coronal CECT in a different patient shows a similar-appearing large mass arising from the right kidney.

INFECTION

Appendicitis

Description: Appendicitis is the inflammation of the vermiform appendix due to an obstruction. Appendicitis is the most common acute surgical condition of the abdomen.

Etiology: Obstruction of the vermiform appendix.

Epidemiology: Appendicitis can occur at any age and affects males and females equally.

Signs and Symptoms: Patient may present with abdominal pain or tenderness in the right lower quadrant (McBurney point), anorexia, nausea and vomiting, and constipation.

Imaging Characteristics: CT examination may be performed either with or without IV contrast. No oral contrast is needed.

CT
- Dilated, fluid-filled appendix.
- May present with a calcified appendicolith.
- Ring-like enhancement with contrast.
- Associated with periappendiceal inflammation or abscess.

Treatment: Immediate surgical intervention (appendectomy) is required.

Prognosis: Usually uncomplicated course of recovery in non-ruptured appendicitis. If the appendix ruptures, there is a variable degree of morbidity and mortality based on the age of the patient.

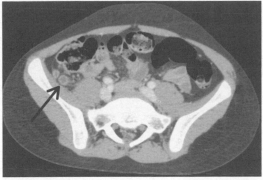

A

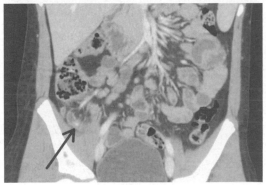

B

FIGURE 1. **Appendicitis.** Axial CECT (A) shows an enlarged rim-enhancing appendix in the right lower quadrant of the abdomen near the cecum with adjacent fat stranding consistent with acute appendicitis. Coronal MPR (B) shows an enlarged enhancing appendix with an appendicolith (*arrow*).

Diverticulitis

Description: Diverticulitis is a complication of diverticulosis. Diverticulitis is an abscess or inflammation initiated by the rupture of the diverticula into the pericolic fat.

Etiology: Diverticulitis is a secondary complication to ruptured diverticula.

Epidemiology: Diverticulosis rarely affects those younger than 40. About 40% to 50% of the general population is affected by the time they reach their sixth to eighth decades of life.

Signs and Symptoms: Pain is most commonly seen in the left lower quadrant. The patient usually experiences either diarrhea or constipation. When considering diverticulitis, in addition to the above, patients will experience fever with chills, anorexia, nausea and vomiting, and tenderness in the left lower quadrant.

Imaging Characteristics:

CT
- Early signs of diverticulitis include wispy, streaky densities in the pericolic fat, and a slight thickening of the colon wall.
- Severe cases of diverticulitis may demonstrate pericolic abscesses.

Treatment: Usually treated with IV antibiotics. Abscess may require CT-guided catheter drainage or surgical intervention.

Prognosis: With early detection and treatment the patient should experience a good recovery.

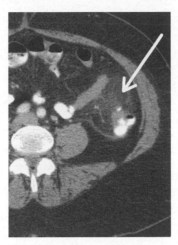

FIGURE 1. **Diverticulitis.** Axial CECT with positive oral contrast shows a moderate amount of fat stranding adjacent to the descending colon on the left due to diverticulitis.

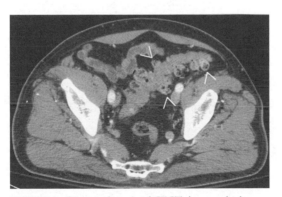

FIGURE 2. **Diverticulitis.** Axial CECT shows multiple diverticula arising from the sigmoid colon, several of which are marked with arrowheads. There is no evidence of acute diverticulitis.

Perinephric Abscess

Description: A perinephric abscess is a collection of pus within the fatty tissue around the kidney.

Etiology: Its results from a bacterial infection such as *E. coli* and *Proteus*, and *Staphylococcus* in a few cases.

Epidemiology: Perinephric abscesses usually arise from a preexisting renal inflammatory disease. However, they may occur as a result of complication of surgery and trauma, or spread from other organs.

Signs and Symptoms: Patients will present with flank or back pain, fever, nausea and vomiting, malaise, and painful urination.

Imaging Characteristics: Contrast-enhanced CT is the modality of choice for the diagnosis.

CT
- Abscess appears with lower than normal attenuation (hypodense) values when compared to normal parenchyma.
- Rim enhancement of the abscess occurs with administration of IV contrast.
- Stranding densities in the perirenal fat and thickening of the renal fascia.
- Gas pockets may be seen within the abscess.

Treatment: Intravenous administration of antibiotics and percutaneous catheter drainage. Surgery is rarely needed.

Prognosis: Generally good with early diagnosis and treatment.

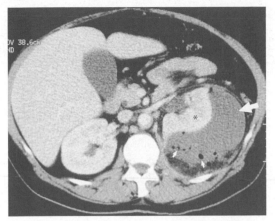

FIGURE 1. **Left Perinephric Abscess.** Contrast CT of the abdomen shows a large fluid collection (*thick arrow*) around the left kidney (*asterisk*). Note: There are gas bubbles within the fluid collection (*small arrows*).

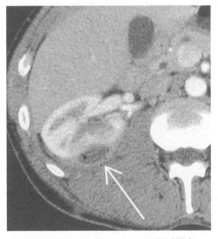

FIGURE 2. **Perinephric Abscess.** CECT shows a rim-enhancing fluid collection adjacent to the right kidney which also contains a few foci of air consistent with a perinephric abscess.

Renal Abscess

Description: A renal abscess is a collection of pus within the parenchyma of the kidney.

Etiology: Results from a bacterial infection.

Epidemiology: Most renal abscesses are the result of an ascending infection and are usually due to gram-negative urinary pathogens, in particular *E. coli*. To a lesser degree, renal abscesses may be due to a complication from surgery, trauma, spread from other organs, or lymphatic spread.

Signs and Symptoms: Patients will present with flank or back pain, fever, nausea and vomiting, malaise, and painful urination.

Imaging Characteristics: Contrast-enhanced CT is the modality of choice for the diagnosis.

CT
- Abscess appears with lower than normal attenuation (hypodense) values when compared to normal parenchyma.
- Rim enhancement of the abscess occurs with administration of IV contrast.
- Stranding densities in the perirenal fat and thickening of the renal fascia.
- Gas pockets may be seen within the abscess.

Treatment: Intravenous administration of antibiotics and percutaneous catheter drainage. Surgery is rarely needed.

Prognosis: Generally good with early diagnosis and treatment.

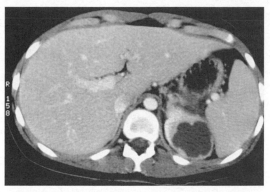

FIGURE 1. **Left Renal Abscess.** CT of the abdomen with IV contrast demonstrates a round low-density mass in the upper pole of the left kidney. Ultrasound showed this mass to be complex. Combination of these findings in a patient with flank pain, fever, and leukocytosis is consistent with a renal abscess.

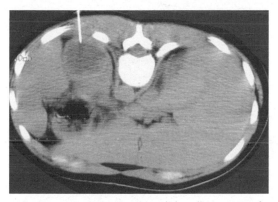

FIGURE 2. **Renal Abscess.** CT-guided needle aspiration of a cystic mass in the upper pole of the left kidney yielded pus. The aspirating needle is within the abscess. This abscess was successfully treated with catheter drainage and antibiotics.

TRAUMA

Liver Laceration

Description: Lacerations to the liver can occur as a result of blunt or penetrating abdominal trauma, as a complication of surgery, or an interventional procedure.

Etiology: A laceration to the liver usually results from an injury, such as blunt or penetrating abdominal trauma. However, complication of surgery or an interventional procedure can also result in a laceration-type injury.

Epidemiology: Trauma to the abdomen results in approximately 10% of all traumatic deaths. Many of these injuries occur as secondary injuries as a result of high-speed motor vehicle accidents.

Signs and Symptoms: Abdominal pain resulting from the blunt trauma or an open wound occurring from a penetrating injury. The patient may experience hypovolemic shock that is caused from an inadequate blood volume.

Imaging Characteristics: CT with IV contrast is the imaging modality of choice in the evaluation of abdominal trauma.

CT
- A noncontrast study may not reveal the injury.
- Contrast enhancement will assist in demonstrating the laceration as a hypodense area.
- May show subcapsular hematoma.
- May show hemoperitoneum.

Treatment: Emergency surgical intervention may be required to repair the laceration of the liver in hemodynamically unstable patients. Stable patients with small lacerations can be treated conservatively.

Prognosis: Depends on the severity of the injury and associated injuries to other organs.

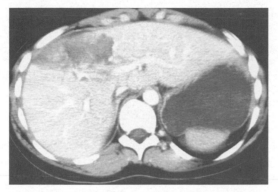

FIGURE 1. **Liver Laceration.** CT of the abdomen with IV contrast demonstrates a large hypodense area of the anterior aspect of the right lobe of the liver consistent with a laceration and hematoma.

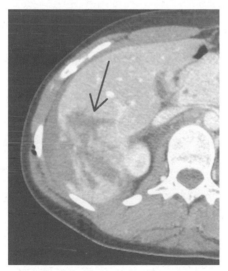

FIGURE 2. **Liver Laceration.** Axial CECT shows jagged linear low-attenuation areas within the right lobe of the liver (*arrow*) with associated blood around the liver consistent with a liver laceration.

Renal Laceration

Description: Laceration of the kidney.

Etiology: Penetrating or blunt trauma to abdomen. Multiorgan involvement occurs in about 75% to 80% of patients who experience penetrating or blunt trauma.

Epidemiology: Renal trauma occurs in about 8% to 10% of patients with significant blunt or penetrating abdominal trauma. Motor vehicle accidents are the most common cause of blunt abdominal trauma. Falls, assaults, including penetrating injuries, are less common.

Signs and Symptoms: Hematuria is seen in approximately 95% of all patients. In addition, flank pain, hematoma, fractured lower ribs, and hypotension may also be seen.

Imaging Characteristics:

CT

- CT with IV contrast modality of choice for patient with blunt or penetrating abdominal trauma.
- Can better evaluate organs with three different window settings (soft tissue, lung, and bone).
- Shows other related trauma to abdomen and pelvis.
- Shows active arterial extravasation.
- Shows extent of hematoma (low-density area).
- Used to confirm two kidneys are present if nephrectomy is considered.

MRI

- Useful in diagnosing renal injury.
- Beneficial in imaging when there is a contraindication to iodinated contrast media.

Treatment: Depending on the degree of injury to the kidney, the majority of patients (approximately 85%) will not require surgery. Nonoperative treatment includes monitoring patient recovery and possible percutaneous drainage of perinephric fluid.

Prognosis: Depends on associated injuries.

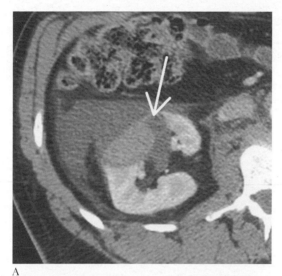

A

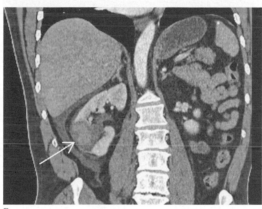

B

FIGURE 1. **Renal Laceration.** Axial (A) and coronal MPR (B) CECTs show a linear hypodense band through the right kidney (*arrow*) with mixed attenuation fluid surrounding the kidney. This is consistent with a renal laceration and associated surrounding hemorrhage and extravasated urine.

Splenic Laceration

Description: The spleen is the most commonly injured abdominal organ. Injury to the spleen can occur as a result of blunt or penetrating trauma to the abdomen.

Etiology: Injuries such as lacerations occur as a result of blunt or penetrating trauma to the abdominal region.

Epidemiology: The spleen is the most commonly injured abdominal organ.

Signs and Symptoms: Depending on the degree of the injury and other related injuries, the patient would probably present with abdominal pain, possible open wound, and symptoms associated with hypovolemic shock (i.e., low blood pressure and rapid pulse).

Imaging Characteristics: CT of the abdomen with IV contrast is the best way to evaluate splenic injuries and also to evaluate other viscera.

CT
- Noncontrast CT may not demonstrate a hematoma or laceration.
- IV contrast CT shows an irregular linear hypodensity of a splenic laceration and perisplenic hematoma. There may also be a hemoperitoneum (blood in the peritoneal cavity).

Treatment: Depending on the extent of the injury, surgical intervention may be required.

Prognosis: Excluding other related injuries that may be associated with the splenic laceration, patient recovery is encouraging.

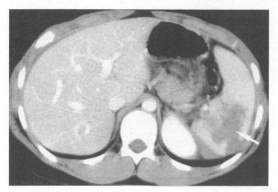

FIGURE 1. Splenic Laceration. CT of the abdomen with IV contrast shows low-density areas (*arrow*) within the posterior aspect of the spleen consistent with a deep laceration and hematomas.

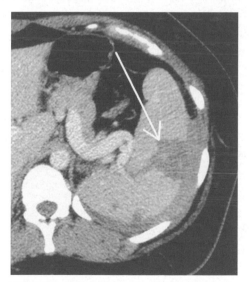

FIGURE 2. Splenic Laceration. Axial CECT shows a jagged low-attenuation area through the spleen (*arrow*) with free fluid surrounding it in a trauma patient. This is characteristic of a splenic laceration.

MISCELLANEOUS

Adrenal Adenoma

Description: An adrenal adenoma is a common benign tumor arising from the cortex of the adrenal gland.

Etiology: These tumors are discovered (incidentally) on an imaging study performed for indications other than adrenal related.

Epidemiology: Adenomas are found in approximately 2% to 9% of autopsies. Since the adrenal gland is the fourth most common site for metastasis (occurring in as many as 25% of patients with a known primary lesion), it is important to determine whether an adrenal mass is benign or malignant.

Signs and Symptoms: Since many adrenal adenomas are incidental finds, they tend to be asymptomatic.

Imaging Characteristics: A normal adrenal gland typically appears in the shape of the letter H, L, Y, T, or V. The adrenal gland is usually about 4 cm in length and 1 cm in width. Adrenal masses are usually an incidental finding. Noncontrast CT, contrast-enhanced CT with washout, and MR with chemical shift imaging are useful in differentiating between adenomas and nonadenomas.

CT
- Appears as a well-circumscribed mass.
- Homogeneous in attenuation and enhancement patterns.
- 10 HU or less (without IV contrast) is a diagnostic indication for adrenal adenoma.
- Relative percentage enhancement washout (RPW) greater than 40% is indicative of a benign tumor.

MRI
- Appears as a well-circumscribed mass.
- Homogeneous signal intensity and enhancement patterns.
- T1- and T2-weighted signal intensity characteristics of adrenal adenomas and adrenal metastases are similar.
- In-phase and out-of-phase imaging is helpful in distinguishing between adenoma and metastases.
- Out-of-phase image of adrenal adenomas show a decrease in signal.

Treatment: Surgery may be performed if tumor is solid, of adrenal origin, and greater than 4 cm in size. Smaller tumor may be monitored periodically to check for growth.

Prognosis: Usually good.

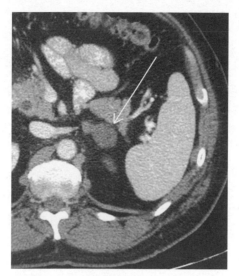

FIGURE 1. Adrenal Adenoma. Axial CECT shows a smooth, well-defined, low-attenuation round mass in the left adrenal gland (*arrow*).

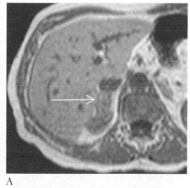

A

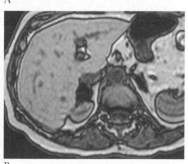

B

FIGURE 2. Adrenal Adenoma. T1W image in phase (A) and out of phase (B) show signal dropout in the right adrenal mass consistent with a fat-containing adrenal adenoma.

Adrenal Metastases

Description: The adrenal gland is the fourth most common site for metastatic spread of disease.

Etiology: Some primary cancers are more likely than others to spread to the adrenal gland. Approximately 50% are melanomas, breast and lung carcinomas comprise about 30% to 40%, and the remaining 10% to 20% are gastrointestinal and renal cell carcinomas.

Epidemiology: Adrenal metastases (at autopsy) are found in up to approximately 30% of cancer patients.

Signs and Symptoms: Adrenal metastases are usually considered to be asymptomatic. With bilateral metastatic involvement, hypoadrenalism may occur. The patient may then present with nonspecific faintness, dizziness, weakness, fatigue, and weight loss.

Imaging Characteristics: Usually bilateral, but may be unilateral. Tumors may vary in size and are less well defined. Larger tumors may have central necrosis and hemorrhages may be seen.

CT
- Typical attenuation of 20 HU or greater on unenhanced examination.
- Below 10 HU indicate benign adenoma on unenhanced examination.

MRI
- T1-weighted images usually demonstrate low to intermediate signal. High signal is seen if hemorrhagic.
- T2-weighted images appear somewhat hyperintense.
- In-phase and out-of-phase imaging is helpful in distinguishing between adenoma and metastases.
- Out-of-phase image of adrenal adenomas shows a decrease in signal.
- Conventional spin-echo and contrast-enhanced MR may not be helpful in determining between benign or malignant tumors.

Treatment: Surgical resection (adrenalectomy) for solitary tumors has contributed to prolonged survival. Radiation therapy may be useful for pain relief. Chemotherapy is not effective for adrenal metastasis.

Prognosis: Fair to poor depending on the extent of spread to other organ systems.

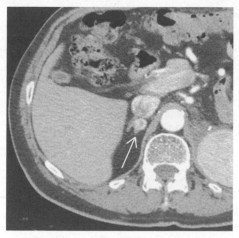

FIGURE 1. **Adrenal Metastases.** Axial CECT
shows a small hyperenhancing right adrenal metastasis
(*arrow*).

Aortic Aneurysm (Stent-Graft)

Description: Stent-grafts have become a promising new catheter-based approach to the repair of abdominal aortic aneurysms (AAA). Interventional radiology is used to place the stent-graft into the normal-diameter aorta above and below the aneurysm, in an effort to isolate the aneurysm from circulation. The stent-graft provides a new, normal-sized lumen to maintain blood flow.

Etiology: The majority of aortic aneurysms occur secondary to atherosclerosis. Other causes include infection, inflammation, trauma, and Marfan syndrome.

Epidemiology: AAA is a relatively common and often fatal condition which primarily affects older patients. With an aging population, the incidence and prevalence of AAA is certain to rise. Approximately 15,000 deaths occur yearly. In 2000, AAA was the 10th leading cause of death in white males 65 to 74 years of age in the United States.

Signs and Symptoms: Most AAAs are asymptomatic. In patients presenting with back, abdominal, or groin pain in the presence of a pulsatile abdominal mass, the aorta should be evaluated.

Imaging Characteristics: Ultrasound may be useful in screening.

CT
- CTA has replaced conventional angiography in preoperative evaluation.
- Less invasive and faster than conventional catheter-based angiography.
- Superior to ultrasound in evaluating rupture or leak.
- Provides 3D images.
- Used to evaluate the placement of the stent-graft.
- Follow-up CT examinations are usually performed at 1, 6, and 12 months, and then yearly to ensure the graft is intact and accomplishing its intended goal.
- Useful to detect and monitor postprocedural complications such as an endoleak, aneurysm enlargement, and graft migration.

MRI
- MRA has 100% sensitivity in detecting aneurysms.
- MRA is useful when there is a contraindication to iodinated IV contrast.

Treatment: An abdominal aortic aneurysm which measures 5 cm or greater in diameter or an aneurysm which has grown from 4 to 5 cm in the past year should be considered for treatment. There are two primary methods for treatment. The traditional open AAA repair method requires direct access to the aorta through an abdominal incision. In the endovascular method, repair of an AAA involves gaining access to the lumen of the abdominal aorta, usually through a small incision over the femoral vessels.

Prognosis: Rupture of an AAA results in a high mortality rate. Morbidity following stent-graft placement is significantly lower than the conventional open surgery.

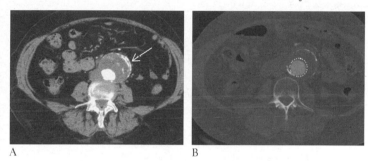

A   B

FIGURE 1. **Aortic Aneurysm.** Axial CECT shows a large abdominal aortic aneurysm with mural thrombus and calcification before (A) and after (B) stent-graft repair.

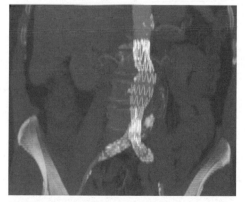

FIGURE 2. **Aortic Aneurysm.** CECT coronal MPR shows an aortoiliac stent-graft.

Hernia: Hiatal Hernia

Description: A condition where part of the stomach protrudes through the esophageal hiatus and enters into the chest cavity. There are two main types: sliding (most common) and paraesophageal.

Etiology: May be either an acquired or a congenital defect. Usually an acquired defect due to decreased abdominal muscle tone and increased pressure within the abdominal cavity. Individuals who are obese, pregnant, have repetitive vomiting issues or are frequently constipated may be more at risk. Aging weakens the elasticity of the esophageal hiatus and may also play a role.

Epidemiology: Frequency increases with age. Majority of individuals are 50 years or older.

Signs and Symptoms: Hiatal hernias cay be asymptomatic and seen as an incidental finding. Larger hiatal hernias may cause heartburn, belching, difficulty in swallowing, pain in the chest or abdominal region, feeling of fullness, or vomiting.

Imaging Characteristics:

CT
- Usually presents as a retrocardiac mass with or without an air-fluid level.

Treatment: While no treatment may be necessary, some individuals may require laparoscopic or minimally invasive surgery.

Prognosis: Good.

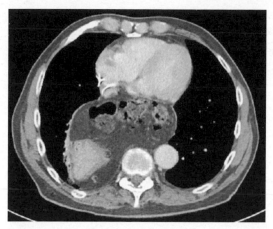

FIGURE 1. **Hiatal Hernia.** Axial CT image shows large retro cardiac hiatal hernia containing portion of the stomach, large bowel, and mesenteric fat.

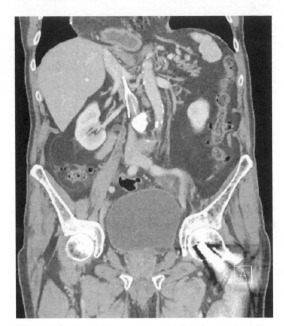

FIGURE 2. **Hiatal Hernia.** Coronal MPR showing bowel in thoracic cavity. Note: IVC filter.

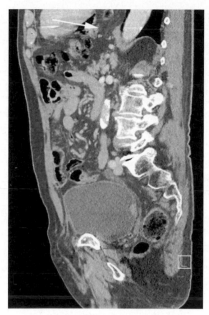

FIGURE 3. **Hiatal Hernia.** Sagittal MPR
showing bowel in thoracic cavity (*arrow*).

Hernia: Inguinal Hernia

Description: A hernia is an abnormal opening or defect through which organs or tissue may protrude through. An inguinal hernia is a hernia in the inguinal (groin area) region of the body. The inguinal hernia is the most common type of abdominal wall hernia. There are two types of inguinal hernias: indirect or direct. Inguinal hernias may occur in children (more commonly indirect type) or adults (both direct and indirect types). Determining whether the specific type of inguinal hernia is indirect (those appearing lateral) or direct (those appearing medial) will depend on their relationship to the inferior epigastric vessels.

In addition to these two types of inguinal hernias, a third hernia (i.e., femoral hernia) may also present in the inguinal (groin area) region.

Etiology: There are two types of inguinal hernias: indirect (congenital) or direct (acquired). Indirect inguinal hernias are more common than the direct type.

Indirect inguinal hernias are associated with a defect in the abdominal wall (internal inguinal ring). This represents an area of potential weakness that the small intestine may protrude through into the inguinal canal and into the scrotum in males. In the female, the hernia follows the course of the round ligament of the uterus to the labia majora. Heavy lifting may also result in an inguinal hernia.

Direct inguinal hernias only occur in males.

Risk Factors: Include incarceration, strangulation, or obstruction of the bowel.

Epidemiology: An inguinal hernia is the most common type of abdominal hernia. Approximately 70% of all inguinal hernias are indirect. Indirect inguinal hernias are more common in males than females with about a 7:1 ratio. Inguinal hernias are more common on the right side than on the left. Direct inguinal hernias only occur in males.

There are more than 1 million abdominal wall hernia surgical repairs performed annually with approximately 750,000 of those being for inguinal hernia repair.

Signs and Symptoms:
- Dull ache or burning pain in the abdomen, groin, or scrotum.
- Bulge or lump in the abdomen, groin, or scrotum. This may be present while coughing or straining and disappear when lying down.

Imaging Characteristics: CT is the gold standard for diagnosis.

CT

◆ A lateral crescent sign. The compression and displacement of the inguinal canal contents such as the vas deferens, testicular vessels, and fat to form a semicircle of tissue that resembles a crescent moon lateral to the hernia. This is useful in diagnosing a direct inguinal hernia.

MRI

◆ Breath-hold or single-shot techniques identify abdominal hernias.
◆ T2-weighted spin-echo.

Treatment: Surgical repair.

Prognosis: Good, depending on the severity of any risk factors that may be present.

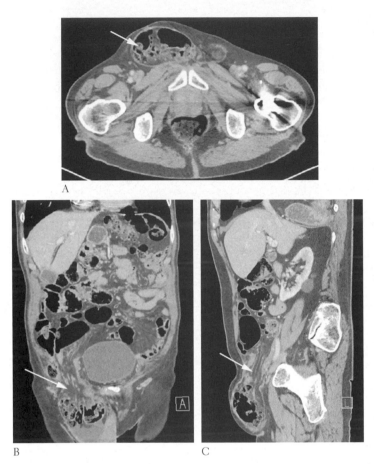

FIGURE 1. **Inguinal Hernia.** (A) Axial CT, (B) coronal MPR, and (C) sagittal MPR showing right inguinal hernia containing bowel (*arrows*).

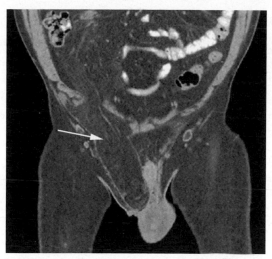

FIGURE 2. **Inguinal Hernia.** Coronal MPR (different case than in Figure 1B) showing only fat in right inguinal hernia (*arrow*).

Hernia: Spigelian Hernia

Description: Spigelian hernia also known as a lateral hernia. The orifice of a Spigelian hernia is located in the Spigelian fascia (aponeurosis), along the lateral border of the abdominal rectus muscle and the transversus abdominis muscle. What is known as the Spigelian hernia belt and where the majority of Spigelian hernias occur is found in a transverse band (approximately 6 cm wide) located between the umbilicus and a line running between both anterior superior iliac spines (ASIS).

The name Spigelian comes from the Belgian anatomist Adrian van den Spieghel who is credited with identifying this uncommon type of hernia.

Etiology: Occurs in a defect in the aponeurosis between the transverse abdominal and rectus abdominal muscles.

Epidemiology: Most commonly occurs between the fourth and seventh decades of life. Usually occurs on the right side. Compared to other hernias, Spigelian hernias tend to be rare. Females are slightly more affected than males.

Signs and Symptoms: Poor bowel function or constipation, dull ache, and recurring pain usually associated with bending or stretching. It does not produce a noticeable bulge in the abdominal wall.

Imaging Characteristics: Herniation may appear to contain bowel or fat.

CT
- CT allows accurate identification of hernias and their contents.
- CT with coronal and sagittal MPRs are very useful in identifying the hernia.
- Good for pre- and postoperative evaluation.

MRI
- Single-shot echo-train spin echo is good in demonstrating hernias.

Treatment: Due to the risk of strangulation, surgery is recommended using a special mesh to strengthen the tissue and prevent reherniation.

Prognosis: Good prognosis following surgical repair with a low risk of reoccurrence.

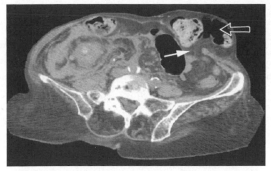

FIGURE 1. **Spigelian Hernia.** Axial CT showing point of herniation through the left abdomen wall (*arrow*) containing a portion of the descending colon (*arrow*). Portion of the descending colon is seen in the hernia sac (*open arrow*).

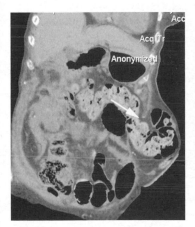

FIGURE 2. **Spigelian Hernia.** Coronal CT MPR showing point of herniation through abdominal wall (*arrow*).

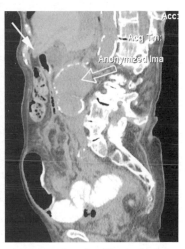

FIGURE 3. **Spigelian Hernia.** Sagittal CT MPR showing point of herniation through abdominal wall (*arrow*). Incidental finding of a large abdominal aortic aneurysm (*open arrow*) is best seen on the sagittal image.

Hernia: Ventral Hernia

Description: Ventral hernias include all hernias involving the anterior and lateral wall of the abdomen. The most common type of ventral hernia is also known as an incisional hernia. An incisional hernia occurs at the site of a previous surgery.

Etiology: May result as either a patient-related or surgery-related factor. Patient-related factors may result from conditions that increase intra-abdominal pressure such as obesity or ascites. Surgery-related factors include the type and location of the incision.

Risk Factors: Large abdominal incision, obesity, diabetes, coughing, heavy lifting, pregnancy, and an increase in pressure due to straining to use the bathroom.

Epidemiology: For incision hernias, approximately 1% to 4% occur after laparotomies, but they occur in 35% to 50% of cases complicated by wound infection or dehiscence. An incisional hernia may occur more than 1 year after surgery; however, most occur within the first 4 months following surgery.

Signs and Symptoms: Protrusion in the abdominal area. Pain may be present especially during physical activity or movement such as when bending forward.

Imaging Characteristics:

CT
- CT allows accurate identification of hernias and their contents.
- CT with coronal and sagittal MPRs are very useful in identifying the hernia.
- Good for pre- and postoperative evaluation.

MRI
- Single-shot echo-train spin echo is good in demonstrating hernias.

Treatment: Surgery is usually the choice of treatment, especially if strangulation is suspected.

Prognosis: Good prognosis following surgical repair with a low risk of reoccurrence.

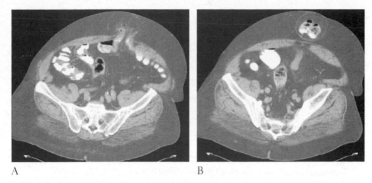

FIGURE 1. **Ventral Hernia.** Axial images of a ventral hernia. (A) Note the site where the intestine is protruding through the abdominal wall. (B) The hernia sac with the intestine is anterior to the abdominal wall.

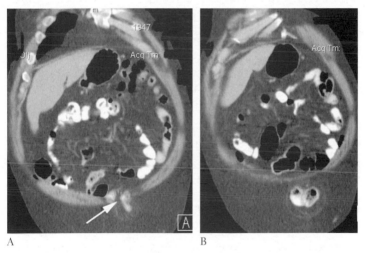

FIGURE 2. **Ventral Hernia.** Coronal MPR of a ventral hernia. (A) Note the site where the intestine is protruding through the abdominal wall (*arrow*). (B) The hernia sac with intestine is outside and anterior to the abdominal wall.

Lymphoma

Description: Lymphomas are malignant tumors involving the lymphatic system. Lymphomas are usually grouped into two groups: (1) Hodgkin disease and (2) non-Hodgkin lymphoma (NHL). As a result of its characteristic pathology (i.e., Reed-Sternberg cell), Hodgkin disease is considered separately. All other malignant lymphomas are grouped under the term non-Hodgkin lymphoma.

Etiology: The cause of malignant lymphomas is unknown; however, viral involvement such as with the Epstein-Barr virus is suspected.

Epidemiology: Approximately 45,000 new cases are diagnosed annually with slightly more than 50% being males. The incidence rises with age, with a median age of 50.

Signs and Symptoms: Similar to Hodgkin disease. Usually involves swelling or enlargement of lymphoid tissue and glands and is painless. Symptoms develop specific to the area involved and systemic complaints of fatigue, malaise, weight loss, fever, and night sweats may be experienced.

Imaging Characteristics: CT is the preferred modality for the diagnosis and staging of lymphoma.

CT
- Used in the staging of lymphomas.
- Can also be used for CT-guided needle biopsies of lymphomas.
- Demonstrates enlarged retroperitoneal, para-aortic, and para-caval lymph nodes.
- Demonstrates enlarged mesenteric lymph nodes.
- Demonstrates enlarged liver and spleen.

Treatment: Radiation therapy and chemotherapy are used to treat non-Hodgkin lymphomas. Surgery is primarily used in establishing the diagnosis and assisting with anatomic staging.

Prognosis: Depends on the cell type and extent of the disease. Hodgkin disease usually has a better prognosis.

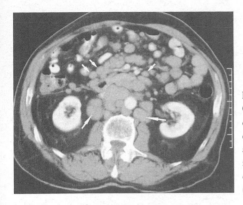

FIGURE 1. Lymphoma.
CT of the abdomen with IV contrast demonstrates multiple enlarged retroperitoneal para-aortic and para-caval lymph nodes (*short arrows*) as well as enlarged mesenteric lymph nodes (*long arrows*).

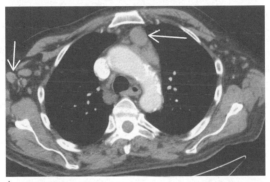

A

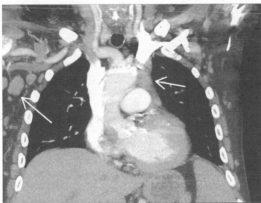

B

FIGURE 2. Lymphoma. CECTs axial (A) and coronal MPR (B) of the chest show bulky mediastinal and axillary lymphadenopathy (*arrows*) in this patient with lymphoma.

Soft-Tissue Sarcoma

Description: Soft-tissue sarcomas of the body consist of a group of malignant tumors that originate in the connective tissues. Sarcomas are named according to the specific type of tissue they affect.

Etiology: It is not known how soft-tissue sarcomas develop. There is some evidence to support that genetics, occupational exposure to certain chemicals such as those found in the agricultural, forestry, railroad, and Vietnam veterans who were exposed to the herbicide agent orange, which contains dioxin, and those with a history of radiation exposure may be more prone to develop soft-tissue sarcomas. There is a latency period associated with the occurrence of soft-tissue sarcomas that seem to exist over the course of several years.

Epidemiology: Soft-tissue sarcomas account for approximately 1% of all malignant tumors found in adults. Roughly 6000 new cases are diagnosed annually with approximately 3300 deaths. Males and females seem to be equally affected. White people are more affected (90%) than black people (6%), and other races contribute to the remaining 4%.

Signs and Symptoms: The signs and symptoms may vary depending on the soft-tissue structure affected. Some patients may present with a palpable mass. Some patients experience pain, while other patients are asymptomatic.

Imaging Characteristics:

CT
- May appear as a solid, mixed, or pseudocystic mass.
- Enhancement with IV contrast may be variable.

MRI
- Signal intensity may be homogeneous or heterogeneous and appear as a mass.
- The type of tissue involved will affect the signal intensity.

Treatment: Surgical intervention with radiation and chemotherapy are used in the treatment of soft-tissue sarcomas.

Prognosis: Depending on the tumor size and anatomical location, histological grade, extent of spread to adjacent tissues and distant metastases, the 5-year survival rate ranges from 30% to 90%. As with all malignant tumors, the prognosis is better with early detection and treatment of the cancer.

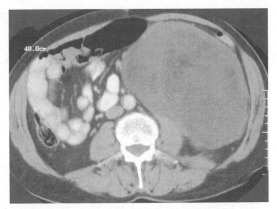

FIGURE 1. Soft-Tissue Sarcoma. Contrast-enhanced CT of the abdomen shows large soft-tissue mass occupying most of the left abdomen displacing bowel loops to the right. There is no significant contrast enhancement.

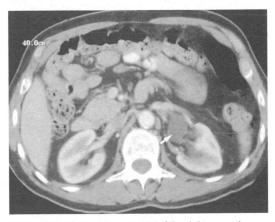

FIGURE 2. Hydronephrosis. CT of the abdomen with contrast shows hydronephrosis of the left kidney (*arrow*) secondary to obstruction of the left distal ureter by the left-sided abdominal mass.

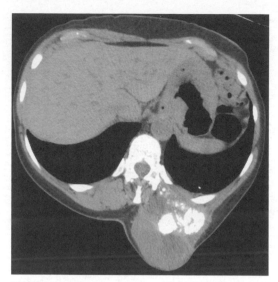

FIGURE 3. **Soft-Tissue Sarcoma.** Axial NECT shows a large soft-tissue sarcoma with areas of low-attenuation central necrosis and coarse dense calcifications arising from the left paraspinal muscles.

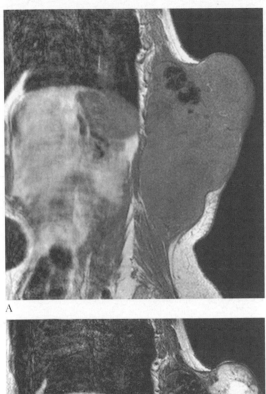

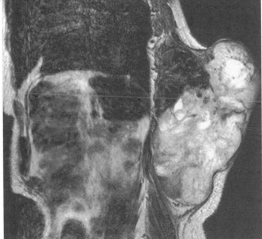

FIGURE 4. **Soft-Tissue Sarcoma.** Sagittal T1W image (A) shows the large posterior paraspinal soft-tissue sarcoma with hypointense calcifications. Sagittal T2W image (B) shows multiple hyperintense areas of necrosis.

Splenomegaly

Description: Splenomegaly is an abnormal enlargement of the spleen.

Etiology: Splenomegaly may be associated with numerous conditions such as a neoplasm, abscess, cyst, infection, portal hypertension (cirrhosis), and hematologic disorders (hemolytic anemia and leukemia).

Epidemiology: Patients with any of the above conditions may develop an enlarged spleen.

Signs and Symptoms: Depends on the causative agent. A palpable mass may be detected in some cases, while splenomegaly may be an incidental finding.

Imaging Characteristics:

CT and MRI
- Shows enlarged spleen.
- Focal lesions may be present.
- Displacement of adjacent organs may be seen.

Treatment: Depends on the causative agent. Surgery may be required.

Prognosis: Depends on the etiology.

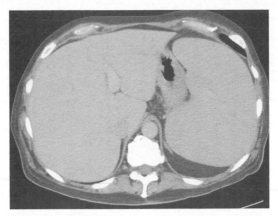

FIGURE 1. **Splenomegaly.** Axial NECT shows an enlarged spleen in a patient with secondary hemochromatosis.

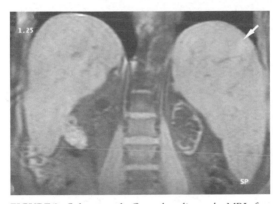

FIGURE 2. **Splenomegaly.** Coronal gradient-echo MRI of the abdomen demonstrates an enlarged spleen (*arrow*).

PART VII

Pelvis

Adenomyosis

Description: Adenomyosis is the presence of endometrium inside the myometrium.

Etiology: Adenomyosis is most likely a result of direct invasion of the endometrium into the myometrium.

Epidemiology: The exact incidence rate is unknown. It is most commonly detected during the fifth decade of life. Adenomyosis is present in 8% to 20% of hysterectomy specimens.

Signs and Symptoms: Patient presents with pelvic pain, menorrhagia, an enlarged uterus, or a combination of the above. Some patients may be asymptomatic.

Imaging Characteristics: MRI is the imaging modality of choice for the diagnosis of adenomyosis. Historically, prior to MRI, adenomyosis was diagnosed by hysterectomy.

MRI
- Thickening either even or uneven (>1 cm) of the junctional zone (JZ).
- Low-signal intensity on T1- and T2-weighted images.
- T1-weighted (T1W) images may show small high-signal intensities representing small foci of hemorrhage.
- T2-weighted images show ill-defined, poorly marginated area of low-signal intensity within the myometrium but contiguous with the JZ.

Treatment: A hysterectomy is the treatment of choice.

Prognosis: Good; this is a benign lesion.

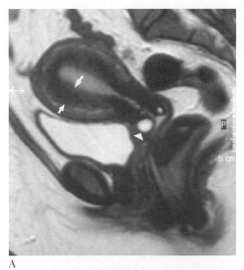

A

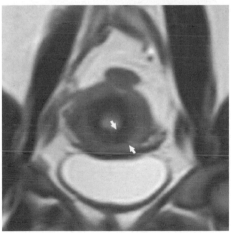

B

FIGURE 1. **Adenomyosis.** T2-weighted sagittal (A) and axial (B) images demonstrate (1 cm) thickening of the junctional (*dark area*) zone (*arrows*) surrounding the endometrial cavity (*bright area*) consistent with adenomyosis. Incidental finding of a nabothian cyst of the cervix (*arrowhead*).

Benign Prostatic Hyperplasia

Description: Benign prostatic hyperplasia (BPH) is a nodular enlargement of the prostate with constriction of the urethra and obstruction of the bladder while emptying.

Etiology: The actual cause is unknown. Some factors such as age and testicles may play a role in the growth of the prostate gland. If the testicles are removed at an earlier age (e.g., for testicular cancer) the man will not develop BPH.

Epidemiology: This is one of the most commonly diagnosed urinary disorders affecting men. About 50% of men between 50 and 60 years of age have histologic evidence of BPH.

Signs and Symptoms: Decrease in the force of the urine stream. Other symptoms may include urinary frequency, urgency, nocturia, intermittent urine flow, incomplete bladder emptying, and straining with urination.

Imaging Characteristics: BPH can mimic prostate cancer.

CT
- Enlarged prostate with a lobulated contour.
- High- and low-density areas within the prostate with variable enhancement.
- Calcification is commonly seen within the prostate.
- Prostate is elevated upward into the bladder.
- Bladder wall thickening.

MRI
- T1-weighted image appears low to intermediate signal.
- T2-weighted image appears intermediate to high signal.
- Difficult to distinguish between BPH and prostate cancer.
- Gadolinium enhancement may be slower and more heterogeneous than prostate cancer.

Treatment: In an acute emergent situation, a catheter is needed to empty the bladder. For patients with symptomatic BPH, a variety of treatment options are available from monitoring to prescribed medications to a variety of surgeries. The surgical "gold standard" is the transurethral resection (TUR).

Prognosis: BPH is benign.

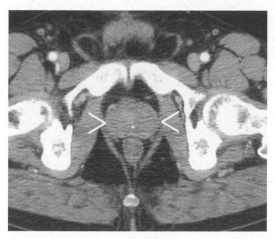

FIGURE 1. **Benign Prostatic Hyperplasia.** Axial contrast-enhanced CT (CECT) shows a heterogeneously enhancing prostate with a small calcification consistent with benign prostatic hyperplasia.

Bladder Cancer

Description: Bladder cancer commonly begins in the innermost lining of the bladder wall called the urothelium or transitional epithelium. Urothelial carcinoma, also known as transitional cell carcinoma (TCC), is the most common type (greater than 90%) of cancer affecting the bladder. Squamous cell carcinoma accounts for about 3% to 8%, while adenocarcinomas make up the remaining 1% to 2% of all bladder cancers.

Tumors may be defined as either noninvasive or invasive. Bladder cancers may also be described as either papillary or flat depending on their appearance.

Etiology: In addition to an increase in age, other risk factors include smoking tobacco, occupational chemical exposure, diet (fried food), certain medications, pelvic radiation, certain Chinese herbs, and genetic mutations.

Epidemiology: Approximately 80,000 new cases are estimated in 2017 with an estimated number of deaths of approximately 17,000. Males are about three times more likely affected than females. Whites are more commonly affected than other races.

Signs and Symptoms: Most common sign is blood in the urine. Pain or burning during urination without evidence of a urinary tract infection. Change in bladder habits.

Imaging Characteristics: The urothelial cells line the urinary tract from the kidney to the urethra, so the entire urinary tract needs to be evaluated for spread of cancer. Cystoscopy is the most useful method to diagnose.

CT
- Useful to detect mass and other abnormalities.
- Renal CT urogram.
- Useful to evaluate pelvis and retroperitoneal lymph nodes.

MRI
MR lymphangiography may be helpful in differentiating inflammatory versus malignant lymph nodes.

Treatment: Clinical staging of the primary tumor is determined by a transurethral resection of the bladder tumor (TURBT). Depending on the stage, the method of treatment may vary. Chemotherapy options may include intravesical or intravenous injection of cancer fighting drugs. Chemotherapy may be administered adjuvant or neoadjuvant. Radiation therapy may be applied externally or internally (brachytherapy) as part of a combined modality therapy. Surgery may range from a transurethral resection (TUR) to a radial cystectomy.

Prognosis: Depends greatly on the stage of the cancer. Patients with a low-stage cancer have nearly a 90% 5-year survival rate. Individuals with high-stage cancer that has invaded into the bladder muscular wall and spread to other organs have a poorer prognosis.

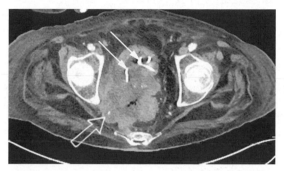

FIGURE 1. **Bladder Cancer.** Axial CT with contrast enhancement. The bladder wall is thickened. There is a lobular soft-tissue mass in the right posterior pelvis encasing the right internal iliac artery (*open arrow*). Bilateral ureteral stents are seen (*arrows*).

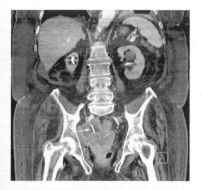

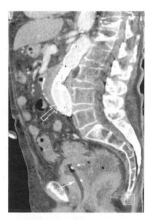

FIGURE 2. **Bladder Cancer.** Coronal MPR CT (same patient as in Figure 1). Note the ureteral stent surrounded by the thickened bladder wall (*arrow*). A small atrophic right kidney is seen also.

FIGURE 3. **Bladder Cancer.** Sagittal MPR CT (same patient as in Figure 1). Note the Foley catheter in urinary bladder (*arrow*). An incidental finding of an AAA is seen (*open arrow*).

Cervical Cancer

Description: Usually slow to develop, the normal cells of the cervix gradually change to a precancerous stage and then if undetected may advance into cervical cancer. Approximately 80% to 90% of cervical carcinomas are squamous cell carcinomas. Most of the remaining cancers (5% to 20%) are adenocarcinomas, which seem to be increasing in frequency particularly among women in their 20s and 30s. Less common types of cervical cancer have a mixed cellular (adenosquamous carcinoma) composition.

Early detection with a Pap test and treatment of precancerous changes can help prevent cancer from developing.

Etiology: Human papillomavirus (HPV) is the most common cause of all cervical cancers. Other causes include multiple sexual partners, smoking, oral contraceptives, weak immune system, overweight, coitus at a young age, pregnancy at an early age, and family history.

Epidemiology: Nearly 13,000 new cases are estimated in 2016 with an estimated number of deaths at about 4100. Cervical cancer is most frequently diagnosed between 35 and 44 years of age. Most women diagnosed with precancerous changes are in their 20s and 30s.

The incidence rate of black Americans is about 30% higher than that of white Americans.

Signs and Symptoms: The most common symptom is an abnormal vaginal bleeding. An abnormal vaginal discharge may also occur.

Imaging Characteristics: MR is the most accurate noninvasive modality for staging.

MRI
- Multiplanar T2-weighted is the main sequence for staging.
- Double oblique technique used to image along the axis of the cervix on the basis of the sagittal and coronal images. This produces true sagittal and axial oblique images of the uterus.
- Dynamic contrast-enhanced imaging may help detect small cervical tumors.
- Diffusion-weighted imaging (DWI) is of little value in staging, however, it is used to locate small cervical tumors in conjunction with T2-weighted imaging.
- 3D T2-weighted fast spin-echo (FSE) or turbo spin-echo (TSE) produces images with increased SNR and CNR, and spatial resolution.
- Vaginal gel is optional. Approximately 20 to 30 mL of warm ultrasonographic gel is placed in the vagina after positioning the patient on the table. When used, the gel produces a high signal on T2-weighted images and provides good detail of the vaginal fornices and cervix.

CT

◆ Most commonly used to evaluate extent and spread of cervical cancer.
◆ CT/PET good to assess distant metastatic disease.
◆ Useful in follow-up evaluation.

Treatment: Depending on the stage, tumor size, histologic features, evidence of metastasis, a combination of surgical procedures, radiation therapy, and chemotherapy options are available.

Prognosis: Precancerous or early cancerous changes, if detected and treated early, have a very good survival rate of approximately 100%. Five-year survival rates vary, 92% for stage I and approximately 20% for stage IV.

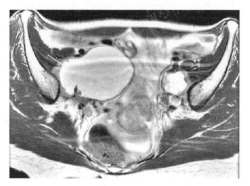

FIGURE 1. Cervical Cancer. Axial T2-weighted image showing mass in the cervical region (*large arrow*). Left and right ovarian cystic structure is present (*small arrows*).

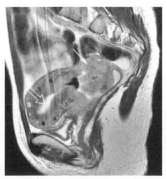

FIGURE 2. Cervical Cancer. Sagittal T2-weighted image showing mass in the cervical region (*arrow*). Fluid collection (*open arrow*) is seen in the uterine cavity secondary to obstructing cervical neoplasm.

Ovarian Carcinoma

Description: Ovarian cancer arises primarily from epithelial tissue.

Etiology: Unknown.

Epidemiology: Occurs between the ages of 30 and 70 years, however, the peak is 59. Ovarian cancer is the second most common gynecologic malignancy and ranks as the fifth most common cancer affecting women. About 10% to 15% of ovarian malignancies are metastases, usually from primary tumors of the GI tract and breast cancer.

Signs and Symptoms: This cancer tends to be asymptomatic and disseminates outside the pelvis early. Vague abdominal discomfort, dyspepsia, flatulence, bloating, and digestive disturbances may be detected early. Late symptoms include abdominal distention and pain, abdominal and pelvic mass, or ascites.

Imaging Characteristics:

CT
- Shows unilateral or bilateral solid and cystic mass.
- Shows multi-lobulated lesion with thick (>3 mm) sometimes irregular enhancing septations.
- Shows ascites.
- Shows enlarged lymph nodes.
- May be used for staging.
- Useful for follow-up to monitor response to therapy and postoperative recurrence.

MRI
- May be used for staging when CT is contraindicated (e.g., pregnancy, use of contrast agents).
- Axial and coronal imaging planes are most useful.

Treatment: Surgery is usually performed for initial staging. Surgery and adjuvant chemotherapy is used in the majority of cases.

Prognosis: The 5-year survival rate drops from 93% in patients with local disease to 28% in those with distant metastases.

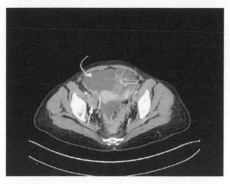

FIGURE 1. Ovarian Cancer. CT axial image shows large multiloculated mass (*curved arrow*) extending from the pelvis into the lower abdominal region with malignant ascites (*open arrow*). Note the right iliac lymphadenopathy (*straight arrow*).

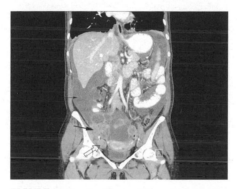

FIGURE 2. Ovarian Cancer. CT coronal MPR shows ovarian tumor (*large black arrow*), large area of ascites (*small black arrow*), and iliac lymphadenopathy on the right side (*open arrow*).

Ovarian Cyst

Description: An adnexal mass of the uterus can comprise any of the appendages of the uterus including the ovaries, fallopian tubes, and the ligaments that hold the uterus in place. The majority of cysts and tumors affecting the ovaries are benign, well circumscribed, round, near-water density with a cyst wall that is difficult to see.

Etiology: Generally related to hormonal dysfunction; however, may be stimulated by other disease processes.

Epidemiology: Occurs more commonly in menarcheal women.

Signs and Symptoms: Adnexal cysts are usually asymptomatic.

Imaging Characteristics: Ultrasound is the best modality for imaging of the uterus and ovaries.

CT
- Contrast-enhanced CT demonstrates a cystic mass in the adnexal region.
- Well-defined margins with fluid density.

MRI
- T1-weighted image shows the cyst with low-signal intensity.
- T2-weighted image shows the cyst with high-signal intensity.

Treatment: Surgery may be required for larger (>5 cm) cysts.

Prognosis: Good; this is a benign cyst.

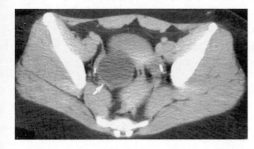

FIGURE 1. **Right Ovarian Cyst.** CT of the pelvis with contrast shows an approximate 5-cm, round, well-defined, low-density mass (*arrow*) in the right adnexal consistent with an ovarian cyst.

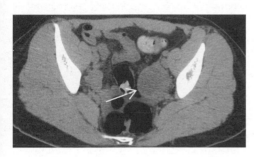

FIGURE 2. **Right Ovarian Cyst.** Axial CT scan demonstrating a cyst on the left ovary.

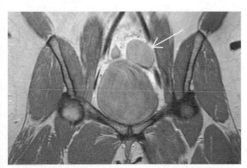

FIGURE 3. **Right Ovarian Cyst.** Coronal T1-weighted MRI showing a left ovarian cyst (*arrow*) which is isointense to water.

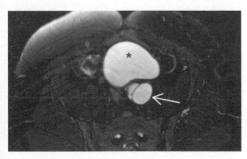

FIGURE 4. **Right Ovarian Cyst.** Axial T2-weighted MRI with an area of increased intensity near the bladder (*asterisk*) corresponding to an ovarian cyst (*arrow*).

Prostate Carcinoma

Description: Prostatic adenocarcinoma is the most common malignancy in males. Prostate cancer affects older males.

Etiology: Unknown. It is suspected there is an inherited or genetic factor involved.

Epidemiology: Typically affects males greater than 50 years of age. This is the third leading cause of cancer deaths in men.

Signs and Symptoms: Screening is useful in detecting asymptomatic cases. Prostate cancer is usually detected during screening with the prostate-specific antigen (PSA) blood test or digital rectal examination (DRE).

Imaging Characteristics:

CT
- Useful for advanced disease.
- Enlarged prostate is common and appears similar to BPH.
- Useful in evaluating lymph nodes and bony anatomy in the abdomen and pelvis.
- CT-guided biopsy useful for directing fine-needle aspiration of enlarged nodes.
- Used for radiation therapy treatment planning.

MRI
- Helpful in problem solving and for staging.
- Use of an endorectal coil may be helpful in staging.

Treatment: Prostate cancer tends to be a slow growing cancer. A "watchful waiting" or "active surveillance" position is suggested to monitor the cancer with regular DRE examinations and PSA tests to see if the cancer is growing. Surgery may be used if the cancer has not spread from the gland. Other methods of treatment such as radiation therapy, cryosurgery, chemotherapy, and a recently Food and Drug Administration (FDA)-approved vaccine sipuleucel-T (Provenge) may be useful.

Prognosis: With early detection and treatment, 5-year survival rate is nearly 100% and 10-year survival rate is in the low 90%.

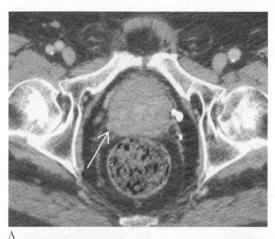

A

B

FIGURE 1. **Prostate Carcinoma.** Axial (A) and sagittal (B)
CECTs demonstrating a heterogeneously enhancing enlarged
prostate (*arrows*) displacing the inferior wall of the bladder
superiorly.

Rectal Cancer

Description: Rectal cancer involves the distance portion of the colon that connects the anus to the large bowel (sigmoid colon). Specifically, the anatomy of the rectum is approximately 15 cm in length and can be divided into three portions (i.e., lower, middle, and upper). Each segment is roughly 5 to 6 cm in length.

Etiology: Usually developing over several years, rectal cancer was initially detected as a precancerous polyp. Some polyps continue to develop into cancer and grow and penetrate the wall of the rectum. Like the colon, the wall of the rectum is comprised of three layers: mucosa (inner layer which is composed of glands that secrete mucus), muscularis (middle layer composed of muscles which help in maintaining its shape and which contract to provide movement of the contents of the bowel), and mesorectum (the fatty tissue surrounding the rectum).

Risk Factors: Include increasing age, smoking, high-fat diet, family history of polyps.

Epidemiology: About 40,000 new cases of rectal cancer detected annually in the United States. About 50% of these cases present as locally advanced disease, defined as T3-4 and/or node-positive in the absence of distant metastases. Males are slightly more affected than females. Individuals 50 and older are more at risk of developing rectal cancer. The most common type of rectal cancer is adenocarcinoma (98%) which arises from the mucosa. Neuroendocrine tumors are the second most common histologic type representing less than 2% of malignant tumors affecting the rectum. From the rectum, cancer can spread to the surrounding lymph nodes and then onto other parts of the body.

Signs and Symptoms: The early stages may not have any symptoms. Symptoms of rectal cancer may include rectal bleeding, blood in the stool, diarrhea or constipation that does not go away, change in the stool, and change in bowel habits, bloating, and change in appetite, weight loss, and fatigue.

Imaging Characteristics: CT of the chest, abdomen, and pelvis is helpful in initial staging and may be beneficial in restaging following neoadjuvant treatment. Accurate reporting of the local-regional extent of the tumor, with specific focus on the anal sphincter area, mesorectal fascia, peritoneum, adjacent organs, and lymph nodes are key. In addition to CT and MR, endorectal ultrasonography may be used to assist with evaluation of the disease. PET/CT may be beneficial in detecting metastatic disease and abdominal lymph nodes. Endorectal ultrasound may be useful in evaluating the extent of local disease (i.e., rectal wall involvement).

CT

* Contrast-enhanced CT of the chest, abdomen, and pelvis for detection of both regional and metastatic disease.
* Useful for follow-up exams.
* Useful in identifying metastases in the lungs and liver.

MRI

* Modality of choice for staging rectal cancer.
* Provides accurate assessment of the mesorectal fascia and sphincter.
* Used to assess local-regional involvement of disease.
* MR is better than CT in detecting local recurrence.
* Conventional T2-weighted and diffusion-weighted imaging (DWI) pre- and posttherapy is beneficial in assessing residual tumor.
* Diffusion-weighted imaging is recommended to R/O liver metastasis.

Treatment: Trimodality approach with neoadjuvant (before surgery) chemotherapy and radiation therapy followed by surgery. Further, the use of adjuvant (after surgery) chemotherapy (AC) in patients with rectal adenocarcinoma who have been treated with surgical resection following neoadjuvant chemoradiation therapy (nCRT) showed an overall survival benefit associated with the additional adjuvant chemotherapy.

Prognosis: Survival rates for rectal cancer have improved as a result of advances in more accurate screening and therapeutic strategies.

The approximate 5-year survival rates are:

- Stage I: 70% to 80%
- Stage II: 50% to 60%
- Stage III: 30% to 40%
- Stage IV: less than 10%

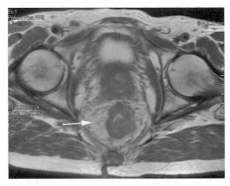

FIGURE 1. **Rectal Cancer.** T2-weighted axial shows large mass on left lateral aspect of the mid to lower rectum (*arrow*).

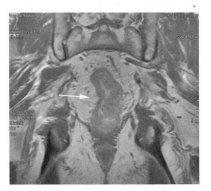

FIGURE 2. **Rectal Cancer.** T2-weighted coronal image shows large mass (about 6 cm in length) on left lateral aspect of the mid to lower rectum (*arrow*).

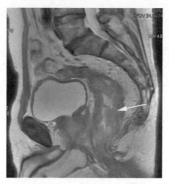

FIGURE 3. Rectal Cancer.
T2-weighted sagittal image shows
large mass in the mid to lower rectum
(*arrow*).

Uterine Leiomyoma (Fibroid Uterus)

Description: Uterine leiomyomas, also known as myomas, fibromyomas, and fibroids, are the most common benign uterine tumors.

Etiology: The cause is unknown. A leiomyoma is an estrogen-dependent tumor that may increase in size during pregnancy, and usually decreases in size following menopause.

Epidemiology: Leiomyomas occur in 20% to 30% of premenopausal women. Black women are affected three times more than white women.

Signs and Symptoms: Depending on the location and size of the tumor, the patient may experience pressure on the surrounding organs and abnormal menstruation.

Imaging Characteristics: Ultrasound is the best imaging modality.

CT
- Usually appear with a homogenous soft-tissue density similar to a normal uterus.
- Calcification may occur in approximately 10% of cases, especially postmenopausal patients.
- Contrast-enhanced images demonstrate enhancement similar to a normal uterus.

MRI
- T1- and T2-weighted images show masses of mixed signal intensity.
- T1-weighted images demonstrate acute hemorrhage as increased signal intensity.
- Multiplanar imaging is very useful for the evaluation of the size and location of the fibroids in the young patient for myomectomy planning.

Treatment: Myomectomy in the young reproductive age group. Hysterectomy for older and severe cases. Uterine artery embolization also may be used to treat the fibroids.

Prognosis: Good; these tumors are benign.

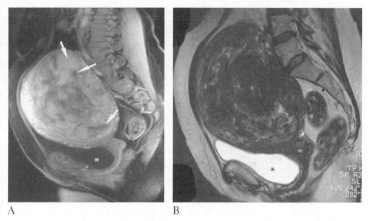

FIGURE 1. Fibroid Uterus. Proton-density (A) and T2-weighted (B) sagittal MR images demonstrate diffusely enlarged uterus compressing the bladder (*asterisk*). There are multiple masses of various signal intensities (*arrows*) of the uterus, seen better on proton-density images.

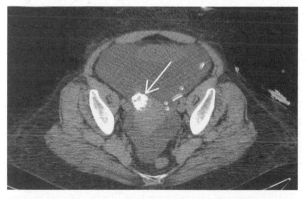

FIGURE 2. Fibroid Uterus. Axial CT showing a densely calcified fibroid.

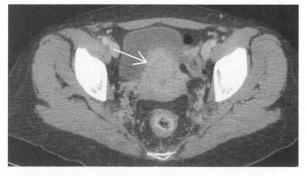

FIGURE 3. Fibroid Uterus. Axial CECT showing a subserosal fibroid.

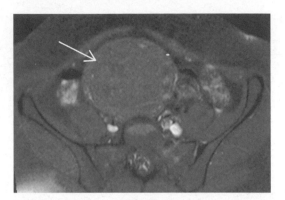

FIGURE 4. Fibroid Uterus. Axial T1W image shows a large fibroid which is isointense to the surrounding uterine muscle.

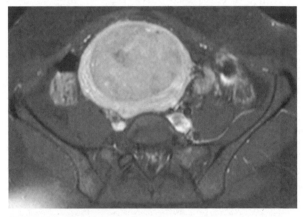

FIGURE 5. Fibroid Uterus. Postcontrast T1W image shows less-intense enhancement of the fibroid compared to the uterus.

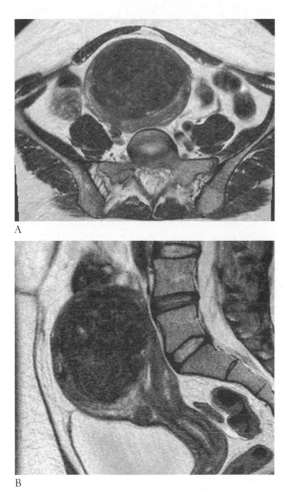

A

B

FIGURE 6. **Fibroid Uterus.** Axial (A) and sagittal (B) T2W images show the large, well-circumscribed transmural fibroid to be hypointense to the uterus.

PART VIII

Musculoskeletal

SHOULDER

Hill-Sachs Fracture (Defect)

Description: A Hill-Sachs fracture is an impaction (compression) fracture of the posterosuperior and lateral aspects of the humeral head. This is usually associated with an anterior dislocation of the shoulder.

Etiology: A Hill-Sachs fracture occurs when the shoulder is traumatically abducted and externally rotated compressing the posterior aspect of the humeral head against the glenoid rim. This force may produce an impaction (compression) fracture of the humeral head characteristic of the injury.

Epidemiology: The associated impaction fracture seen in a Hill-Sachs fracture occurs in approximately 60% of the population diagnosed with an anterior dislocation of the shoulder.

Signs and Symptoms: Pain, stiffness, shoulder instability, avascular necrosis, and posttraumatic myositis ossificans may accompany this injury.

Imaging Characteristics:

CT
- Reveals the compression fracture associated with injury to the posteriolateral aspect of the humeral head resulting from an anterior dislocation of the shoulder. Hill-Sachs fracture is best seen at the level of the coracoid.

MRI
- Appear as wedge-like defects on the posteriolateral aspect of the humeral head.
- T1-weighted (T1W) images show the low-signal injury.
- T2-weighted images depict the injury as hyperintense.
- STIR images are more sensitive for the diagnosis of subtle fracture or bone bruise appears with a high signal.
- MR arthrography is excellent for the evaluation of tears of the glenoid labrum in patients with recurrent shoulder dislocation.

Treatment: Surgical intervention may be required for recurrent shoulder dislocation.

Prognosis: Results may vary depending on extenuating circumstances; however, the patient is encouraged to gradually resume normal use.

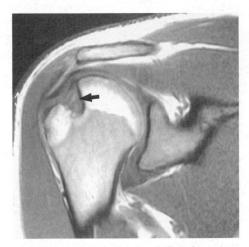

FIGURE 1. **Hill-Sachs Fracture.** Hill-Sachs fracture seen in a patient with a history of an anterior dislocation of the shoulder. T1-weighted oblique coronal image of the shoulder demonstrates a wedge-shaped defect in the superior lateral aspect of the head of the humerus (*arrow*) consistent with a Hill-Sachs fracture.

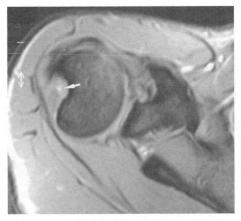

FIGURE 2. **Hill-Sachs Fracture.** Gradient-echo axial image of the shoulder demonstrates a wedge-shaped defect (*arrow*) along the posterior lateral aspect of the head of the humerus consistent with a Hill-Sachs fracture.

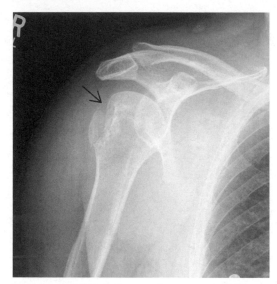

FIGURE 3. Hill-Sachs Fracture. Anteroposterior (AP) shoulder radiograph shows a Hill-Sachs fracture with a deformity of the lateral humeral head and avulsion of the greater tuberosity.

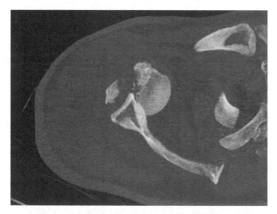

FIGURE 4. Hill-Sachs Fracture. MIP axial CT shows impaction of the anterior glenoid with the humeral head as it is anteriorly dislocated resulting in a Hill-Sachs fracture deformity.

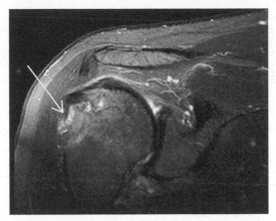

FIGURE 5. **Hill-Sachs Fracture.** Coronal T2W MR image shows a fracture deformity and hyperintense edema in the humeral head consistent with a Hill-Sachs fracture.

Labral Tear

Description: The labrum is a ring of fibrocartilage around the edge of an articular joint such as the glenoid labrum of the shoulder joint and the acetabular labrum of the hip joint. Tearing of the labrum is referred to as a labral tear. Most common labral tears include superior labral antero-posterior (SLAP) tear and a Bankart lesion. A SLAP tear is most commonly seen in overhead throwing type of activities and is located where the biceps tendon attaches to the shoulder. A Bankart lesion is a labral tear that occurs when a shoulder is dislocated.

Etiology: Injuries can result from chronic trauma due to repetitive motion or from acute trauma as result of a fall or heavy lifting.

Epidemiology: The glenoid labrum of the shoulder joint is most commonly affected.

Signs and Symptoms: Pain with overhead motion, at night or with daily activities, decreased range of motion, and loss of strength in the shoulder.

Imaging Characteristics:

CT
- CT arthrography is helpful in detecting labral tears.

MRI
- Oblique coronal plane of the supraspinatus tendon is good to evaluate the rotator cuff.
- Degenerative labra appear as a fuzzy or indistinct surface.
- MR arthrography and MR imaging good to show labral tear.
- MR arthrography good to see detached labral fragment and labral degeneration.
- MR arthrography best to see inferior part of labrum and the inferior glenohumeral ligament.
- Abduction with external rotation (ABER) position is used to better evaluate the inferior glenohumeral ligament.

Treatment: Nonsteroidal anti-inflammatory drugs (NSAIDs) and rest with exercise to strengthen the rotator cuff may be recommended. In more severe cases, arthroscopic surgery may be required.

Prognosis: Usually good recovery is expected in SLAP repairs.

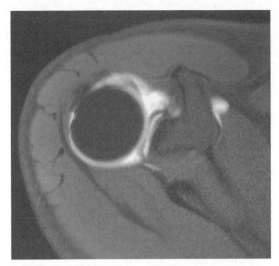

FIGURE 1. **Labral Tear.** Axial MR arthrogram T1W fat-suppressed (FS) image of the shoulder shows a widened, high-signal fluid collection between the glenoid and labrum consistent with a SLAP tear.

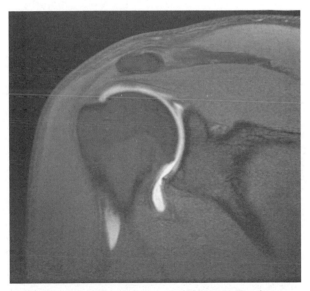

FIGURE 2. **Labral Tear.** Oblique coronal T1W FS MR arthrogram shows high-signal intensity within the superior labrum consistent with a SLAP tear.

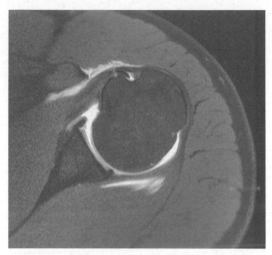

FIGURE 3. Labral Tear. Axial MR arthrogram T1W FS image shows a small hyaline articular cartilage defect with adjacent fraying of the labrum. Glenoid labrum articular disruption (GLAD) lesion refers to an anterioinferior labral tear.

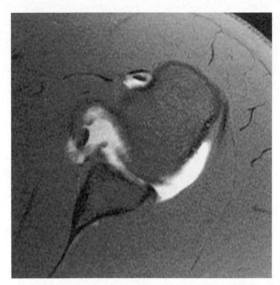

FIGURE 4. **Labral Tear.** Axial MR arthrogram T1W FS image shows a larger hyaline articular cartilage defect with disruption of the labrum. GLAD: Glenoid labrum articular disruption.

Pectoralis Major Tendon Tear

Description: The origin of the pectoralis major muscle is the sternum, clavicle, and cartilages of the 1st to 6th ribs. Its insertion is to the bicipital ridge of the humerus. The pectoralis major muscle action is to flex, adduct, and rotate the arm. Complete or partial tearing may occur.

Etiology: Most commonly caused by forced abduction, external rotation, and extension of the shoulder against resistance. This injury commonly results from bench pressing or weightlifting, wrestling, an altercation, pulling, football, or a fall. More commonly seen in men and high-performance athletes.

Epidemiology: Ruptures of the pectoralis major tendon are relatively uncommon. Injuries may be classified as either acute (<8 weeks from injury) or chronic (>8 weeks from injury).

Signs and Symptoms: Pain, swelling, decreased range of motion, ecchymosis, and later muscular deformity (muscle retraction) at the site of rupture. Weakness in the shoulder adduction and internal rotation is present.

Imaging Characteristics: MRI preferred choice when evaluating for pectoralis major tendon tear.

As a side note, performing a routine shoulder is not optimal for evaluation of the pectoralis major. A larger FOV and RF coil are needed. Further, the referring physician should indicate clearly that the desired MRI is of the chest wall or upper extremity searching for pectoralis major tear rather than a shoulder MRI.

CT

- In severe trauma situation where shoulder prosthesis is considered, CT is helpful in evaluating the relationship between the glenoid and the pectoralis major muscle (essential marker for implantation of a humeral component) for preoperative planning.

MRI

- Shows intramuscular and perimuscular edema of the pectoralis major muscle, muscle retraction, and absence of a normal humeral insertion.
- T2-weighted images with fat-suppression superior in showing subtle abnormalities, particularly incomplete tears.
- Axial images provide optimal visualization of the muscle and insertion.
- Coronal oblique and sagittal oblique confirm findings of axial plane imaging.
- Useful for surgical planning by (1) determining the exact location of the injury; and (2) degree of rupture.

Treatment: Surgery followed with physical therapy.

Prognosis: Early surgical repair shows better outcome than delayed repair.

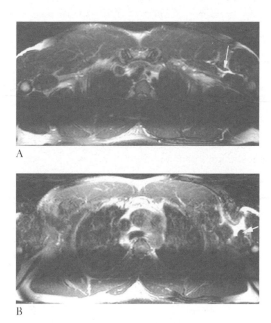

FIGURE 1. **Pectoralis Major Tendon Tear.** MRI axial T2-weighted adjacent images show complete tear of the left pectoralis tendon near the humerus (*arrow*). Note: High signal surrounding complete tear.

Rotator Cuff Tear

Description: The rotator cuff of the shoulder is comprised of a thick, tough, tendinous capsule surrounding the four tendons representing the insertions of the supraspinatus, infraspinatus, the teres minor muscles (insert into the greater tuberosity and assist with external rotation), and the subscapularis (inserts into the lesser tuberosity and assists with internal rotation). Tearing of the rotator cuff can be categorized as partial or complete tears.

Etiology: Usually results from chronic degenerative impingement. Other causes may include acute and chronic trauma. Sports and occupational overuse may also be associated with rotator cuff tears.

Epidemiology: Injury involving the rotator cuff is one of the most common causes of shoulder pain and disability.

Signs and Symptoms: Progressive pain and weakness accompanying a loss of motion. Shoulder pain increases when performing activities at or above the level of the shoulder. Night pain is often experienced.

Imaging Characteristics: MRI has completely replaced shoulder arthrography.

MRI
- T2-weighted fat-saturated images show the tear as high signal.
- There may be discontinuity and retraction of the rotator cuff tendons.
- Fluid in the subacromial/subdeltoid bursa.
- Superior migration of the head of the humerus.
- Degenerative hypertrophy of the acromioclavicular (AC) joint.
- MR arthrography is also useful for the evaluation of labral tears.

Treatment: Depends on the severity of the injury. Early diagnosis, pain management, and surgical intervention may encourage better patient outcome.

Prognosis: Patient outcome varies depending on the degree of the injury, method of treatment, patient discomfort level with pain, and shoulder mobility.

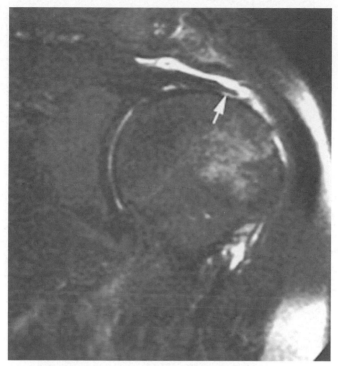

FIGURE 1. **Rotator Cuff Tear.** T2-weighted oblique coronal MRI with fat suppression shows a full-thickness tear (*arrow*) of the distal rotator cuff tendon (supraspinatus muscle) with some medial retraction. A small amount of fluid is in the subacromial/subdeltoid bursa.

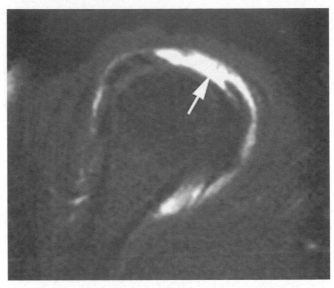

FIGURE 2. Rotator Cuff Tear. Fat-suppressed T2-weighted oblique sagittal image demonstrates a full-thickness tear (*arrow*) of the rotator cuff with fluid in the subacromial/subdeltoid bursa.

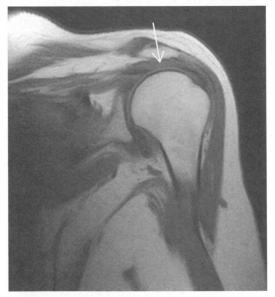

FIGURE 3. Rotator Cuff Tear. T1-weighted coronal spin-echo MR shows disruption of the hypointense supraspinatus tendon.

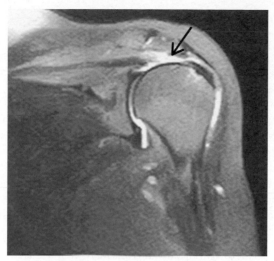

FIGURE 4. Rotator Cuff Tear. Coronal FS T2W image shows a full-thickness tear of the supraspinatus tendon with moderate retraction.

ELBOW

Biceps Brachii Tendon Tear

Description: The bicep brachii muscle is located on the anterior side of the upper arm. The proximal end of the biceps brachii muscle has two tendons, the long head that passes through the bicipital groove and attaches to the glenoid and the short head that attaches to the coracoid process of the scapula. The distal end insertion is the bicipital tuberosity of the radius. The biceps brachii muscle action is to flex the arm and forearm and to supinate the hand. Ruptures of the bicep brachii tendon can be classified as either partial or complete.

Etiology: There are two main causes for biceps tendon tears: injury and overuse. Specifically, the distal biceps brachii tendon tear is complete and is usually the result of a single traumatic event.

Risk factors include: Increasing age, heavy overhead activities, lifting a heavy weight, overuse, smoking (nicotine affects nutrition), and corticosteroid medications. Overuse can cause other shoulder-related problems such as tendinitis, shoulder impingement, which may contribute to weakening or tearing of the rotator cuff.

Epidemiology: Ruptures of the proximal biceps brachii tendon comprise about 90% to 97% of all biceps ruptures and almost exclusively involve the long head. Remaining ruptures occur distally at the insertion on the radial tuberosity, or even less common, at the short head insertion on the coracoid.

- Individuals between 40 and 60 years of age with a history of shoulder problems, secondary to chronic wear. Younger individuals may rupture the biceps brachii tendon due to trauma.
- Males are more commonly affected than females, primarily due to occupational factors.

Signs and Symptoms: A torn tendon may result in a bulge (Popeye muscle) in the upper arm. Additional signs and symptoms may include:

- Sudden sharp pain at the site of the tear.
- An audible pop or snapping sound.
- Bruising from the middle of the upper arm down toward the elbow on the medial side.
- Cramping of the bicep muscle with use.
- Weakness.
- Difficulty in supinating or pronating the hand.

Imaging Characteristics:

MRI

- T2-weighted fat-saturated and proton-density weighted images show high-fluid signal surrounding retracted tear (low signal) of the biceps tendon.

Treatment: Depending on the extent of the injury, nonsurgical treatment may include ice, nonsteroidal anti-inflammatory medication, rest, and physical therapy. Surgical treatment of a bicep tendon tear is rarely performed. Successful surgical outcome can correct the Popeye muscle deformity and restore strength and function to near-normal status.

Prognosis: Patient outcome varies depending on the degree of the injury.

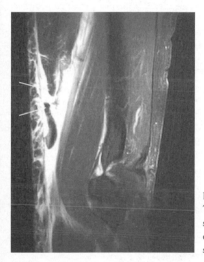

FIGURE 1. Biceps Brachii Tendon Tear. Sagittal T2-weighted SPAIR image showing a complete tear and retraction of the bicep tendon (*arrows*) with surrounding edema.

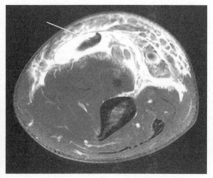

FIGURE 2. Biceps Brachii Tendon Tear. Axial T2-weighted SPAIR image showing retracted bicep tendon (*arrow*) with surrounding edema.

Triceps Tendon Tear

Description: The triceps tendon is the least common of all tendons in the body to rupture and is an uncommon cause of posterior elbow pain. Tearing of the triceps tendon can be classified as partial or complete. A complete tearing of the triceps tendon is not common and partial tears are even less common. The tendon will typically rupture at its attachment near the olecranon.

Etiology: A rupture of the triceps tendon usually occurs as a result of direct blow to the tendon, a fall on an outstretched arm, or a decelerating counterforce during active extension. In some cases, the tendon may undergo degeneration or erosion in association with olecranon bursitis.

Epidemiology: The triceps tendon is the least common of all tendons in the body to rupture.

Signs and Symptoms: Patient presents with posterior elbow pain.

Imaging Characteristics: MRI is the imaging modality of choice.

MRI
- Axial and sagittal imaging is necessary to evaluate partial versus complete tear and size of the gap associated with the tear. This information is useful in preoperative planning.
- Abnormal increased signal may be seen in the tendon in a partial tear or tendinopathy.
- Discontinuous fibers are noted with complete tear.
- Most tears occur at the insertion onto the olecranon.

Treatment: Surgical repair is required as soon as possible.

Prognosis: In general, the results are good.

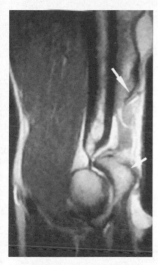

FIGURE 1. **Triceps Tendon Tear.** T2-weighted axial MRI shows increased signal intensity within the distal triceps tendon (*long arrow*) near its insertion to the olecranon process of the ulnar (*short arrow*).

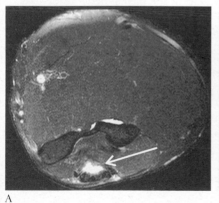

FIGURE 2. **Triceps Tendon Tear.** Sagittal T2-weighted MRI shows a completely torn and retracted triceps tendon (*long arrow*) from the olecranon (*short arrow*).

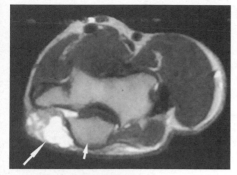

A   B

FIGURE 3. **Triceps Tendon Tear.** Axial (A) and sagittal (B) FS T2W sequences show increased signal in the normally hypointense triceps tendon consistent with a tear and surrounding edema.

HAND AND WRIST

Carpal Tunnel Syndrome

Description: Carpal tunnel syndrome results from a compression of the median nerve in the carpal tunnel.

Etiology: Compression neuropathy of the medial nerve. There appears to be an association with repetitive activity such as typing.

Epidemiology: Most commonly seen in individuals between the ages of 30 and 60 years who perform repetitive actions with their hands and wrist. Though there are several potential factors which may increase the pressure within the carpal tunnel and compress the medial nerve, which then may lead to carpal tunnel syndrome, many cases tend to be idiopathic.

Signs and Symptoms: Tingling and numbness affecting the median nerve distribution of the radial three and one-half (first through third digits and the radial side of the fourth digit) digits. Patients will present with pain, described as deep and aching or throbbing diffusely throughout the hand and radiating up the forearm.

Imaging Characteristics: Imaging may not be required to make the diagnosis. Diagnosis is usually made clinically with the assistance of an electromyogram.

MRI
- May show proximal enlargement of the medial nerve at the level of the pisiform.
- May be beneficial for follow-up evaluation after surgery.

Treatment: Injection of hydrocortisone may benefit most patients if diagnosed early. Surgery is performed to release the flexor retinaculum.

Prognosis: Good.

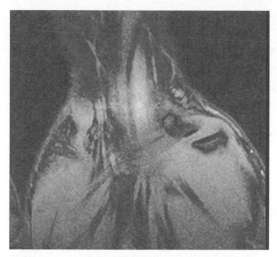

FIGURE 1. Carpal Tunnel Syndrome. Coronal T2W MR of the wrist showing increased signal within the median nerve.

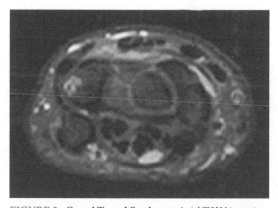

FIGURE 2. Carpal Tunnel Syndrome. Axial T2W inversion recovery MR image of the wrist shows an enlarged and hyperintense median nerve within the carpal tunnel at the level of the pisiform.

Gamekeeper Thumb

Description: Results from an abduction injury to the ulnar collateral ligament of the first (thumb) metacarpophalangeal joint.

Etiology: Forceful radial and palmar abduction of the thumb usually resulting from snow skiing accidents and falls on an outstretched hand.

Epidemiology: Anyone experiencing a forceful radial and palmar abduction of the thumb is at risk.

Signs and Symptoms: Pain, swelling, and ecchymosis around the metacarpophalangeal joint.

Imaging Characteristics:

MRI
- May show avulsion fracture at the attachment site of the ulnar collateral ligament (one-third of cases).
- Shows tear of the ulnar collateral ligament as a thin, low-signal ligament or discontinuity of the ligament with hemorrhage and edema surrounding the torn ends of the ligament.

Treatment: Surgical repair.

Prognosis: Early surgical repair produces better results.

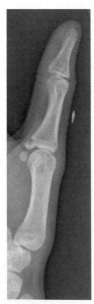

FIGURE 1. **Gamekeeper Thumb.** Lateral radiograph of the thumb shows a small avulsion fracture off the base of the proximal phalanx on the ulnar side at the insertion of the ulnar collateral ligament.

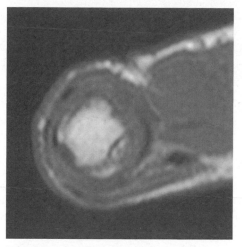

FIGURE 2. **Gamekeeper Thumb.** Axial T1 shows a displaced bone fragment off the base of the first proximal phalanx.

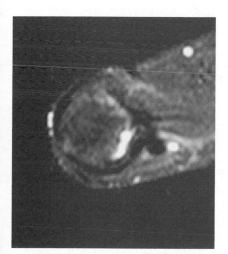

FIGURE 3. **Gamekeeper Thumb.** Axial T2 shows increased signal in this region as a result of edema.

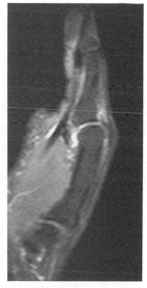

FIGURE 4. **Gamekeeper Thumb.** Coronal proton-density (PD) MR shows a displaced bone fragment and edema at the insertion of the ulnar collateral ligament.

Ganglion Cyst

Description: A ganglion is a small (1.0 to 2.0 cm) benign cyst that may be seen around any joint capsule or tendon sheath. It is commonly located around the joints of the wrist.

Etiology: There is no known cause for the development of ganglions; however, they are suspected to be caused by a coalescence of small cysts formed as a result of degeneration of periarticular connective tissue.

Epidemiology: Ganglions typically present between the second and fourth decades of life. There is a slight female predominance.

Signs and Symptoms: These firm, movable lesions are often asymptomatic. Ganglions that occur in the carpal tunnel or Guyon canal may cause compression of the median and ulnar nerves, respectively.

Imaging Characteristics:

CT
◆ Round, low-density mass with fluid-attenuation value.

MRI
◆ A ganglion is usually a round, lobulated, homogeneous mass with low signal on T1-weighted images.
◆ This cystic lesion will appear hyperintense on T2-weighted images.
◆ Postcontrast T1-weighted images will not enhance.

Treatment: Surgical excision of the ganglion cyst.

Prognosis: Good; this is a benign cyst.

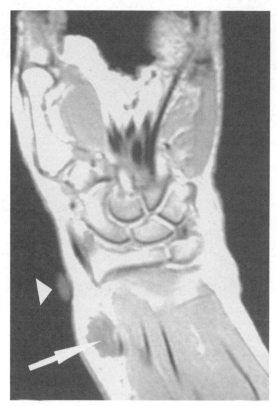

FIGURE 1. **Ganglion Cyst.** T1-weighted coronal image demonstrates a lobulated low-signal-intensity mass (*arrow*) along the radial aspect of the distal forearm. Note: The vitamin E capsule (*arrowhead*) marking the site of the palpable abnormality.

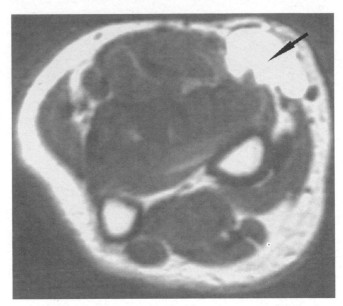

FIGURE 2. **Ganglion Cyst.** T2-weighted image demonstrates a lobulated high-signal-intensity mass (*arrow*) with well-defined margins consistent with a ganglion cyst along the volar radial aspect of the distal forearm close to the wrist.

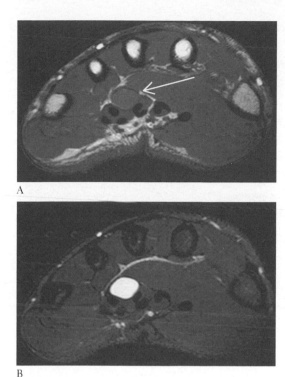

A

B

FIGURE 3. **Ganglion Cyst.** Axial MR images of the hand show a well-circumscribed mass adjacent to the flexor tendons that is dark on T1W (A) and bright on FS T2W (B).

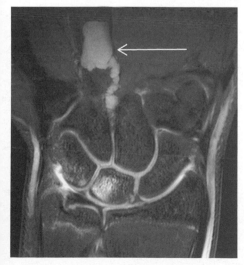

FIGURE 4. **Ganglion Cyst.** Coronal T2W spectral presaturation with inversion recovery (SPIR) shows a ganglion cyst arising from the capitohamate joint.

Kienbock Disease

Description: Is a condition which results in osteonecrosis of the carpal lunate bone.

Etiology: The underlying cause is usually not known; however, osteonecrosis may occur as a result of repetitive trauma (e.g., manual labor or sports related), acute fracture, or ulnar minus variance.

Epidemiology: Usually affects the dominant wrist of men between 20 and 40 years of age.

Signs and Symptoms: Pain which worsens with activity. Swelling and tenderness is usually noted over the radiocarpal joint.

Imaging Characteristics:

MRI
- Coronal plane best for showing anatomy.
- T1- and T2-weighted images show osteonecrosis as low signal.
- Useful in monitoring postsurgical intervention and revascularization.

Treatment: Immobilization and nonsteroidal anti-inflammatory drugs (NSAIDs) are used in less severe cases. Surgical intervention is considered for more advanced cases.

Prognosis: Depends on the severity of the condition.

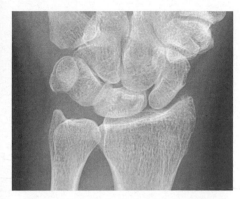

FIGURE 1. Kienbock Disease. AP radiograph of the wrist shows sclerosis of the lunate.

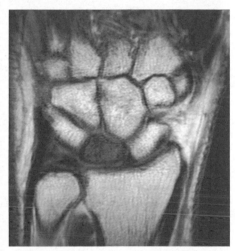

FIGURE 2. Kienbock Disease. T1W coronal MR image of the wrist shows loss of normal marrow signal in the lunate.

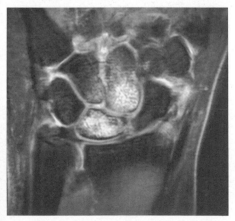

FIGURE 3. Kienbock Disease. Proton-density coronal MR image of the wrist shows increased signal in the lunate and proximal capitate due to edema.

Triangular Fibrocartilage Tear

Description: The triangular fibrocartilage complex (TFCC) is a ligamentous and cartilaginous structure located in the ulnocarpal space of the wrist. The TFCC stabilizes the distal radioulnar joint and ulnar carpus (the joint between the arm and hand, made up of eight carpal bones). Injury to this structure may result in a tear.

Etiology: TFCC tears are associated with a positive ulnar variance. An ulnar variance increases with pronation and grip, and decreases with supination. Injuries may result from the following situations: (1) a fall onto a pronated hyperextended wrist; (2) power-drill injury in which the drill binds and rotates the wrist instead of the bit; (3) distraction force applied to the volar forearm or wrist; or (4) distal radius fracture.

Epidemiology: Anyone experiencing any of the above-listed causes is at risk.

Signs and Symptoms: Injuries to the TFCC present as pain in the ulnar side of the wrist. Weakness and occasional clicking sound is common with an injury.

Imaging Characteristics:

MRI

- Coronal plane is best for showing tear.
- GRE (gradient echo) good for showing anatomy.
- STIR (short-tau inversion recovery) good for showing tears.
- MR arthrography is very helpful in identifying TFCC tears.

Treatment: Conservative treatment consisting of nonsteroidal antiinflammatory drugs (NSAIDs), immobilization, and physical therapy. Surgical intervention may be required for more serious cases.

Prognosis: Depends on the severity of the injury. For less severe injuries, results are usually good.

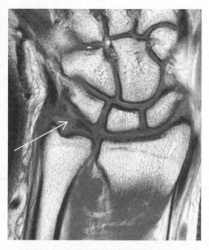

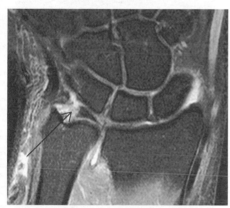

FIGURE 1. **Triangular Fibrocartilage Tear.** Coronal T1W image shows disruption of the TFCC and surrounding edema.

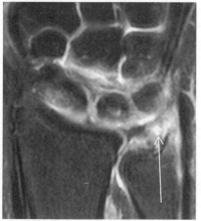

FIGURE 2. **Triangular Fibrocartilage Tear.** Coronal T2W image shows disruption of the TFCC with hyperintense surrounding fluid.

FIGURE 3. **Triangular Fibrocartilage Tear.** Coronal T2W spectral presaturation with inversion recovery (SPIR) shows diffuse hyperintense edema in the region of the TFCC.

HIP

Avascular Necrosis (Osteonecrosis)

Description: Avascular necrosis (AVN) occurs as an interruption in the blood flow within the bone (e.g., femoral head), resulting in the death of the hematopoietic cells, osteocytes, and marrow fat cells making up the bony structure.

Etiology: Avascular necrosis may result from trauma (fractures, dislocation), corticosteroids, caisson disease (in which individuals who are removed too quickly from a high-pressure environment, such as in deep water diving, are prone to develop nitrogen bubbles which may cause a bony infarct), Legg-Calve-Perthes disease, sickle cell disease, or radiation exposure; or it may be idiopathic.

Epidemiology: The hip is the most common site affected. Males are more affected than females by as much as a 4:1 ratio. Most patients diagnosed with AVN are between 30 and 70 years of age. Bilateral involvement may occur in as many as 50% of the cases.

Signs and Symptoms: Increased joint pain as bone and joint begin to collapse, limited range of motion due to pain, decreased usage of the limb involved.

Imaging Characteristics: MRI is the most sensitive modality for the diagnosis of avascular necrosis.

MRI
- Diffuse edema.
- Serpiginous line (low-signal intensity) with a fatty center.
- Focal subchondral low-signal lesion on T1-weighted images and variable signal on T2-weighted images.

Treatment: Treatments may include medications for pain, assistive devices to reduce weight on the bone or joint, core decompression, osteotomy, bone graft, arthroplasty (total joint replacement), electrical stimulation, or any combination of therapies to encourage the growth of new bone.

Prognosis: Mixed and variable, dependent on the underlying cause of the disease, overall health and medical history, extent of the disease, location and amount of bone affected, and tolerance to specific medications, procedures, or therapies.

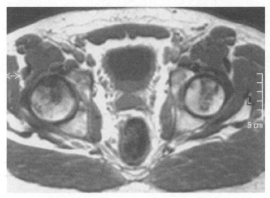

FIGURE 1. Avascular Necrosis of the Femoral Heads.
T1-weighted axial MRI shows focal decreased marrow signal
intensity of the femoral heads bilaterally. The right femoral
head is worse than the left.

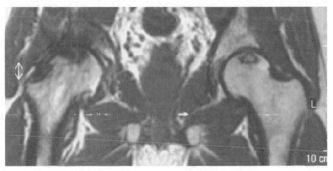

FIGURE 2. Avascular Necrosis of the Femoral Heads. T1-weighted
coronal MRI shows focal decreased marrow signal intensity of the femoral
heads bilaterally, worse on the right side.

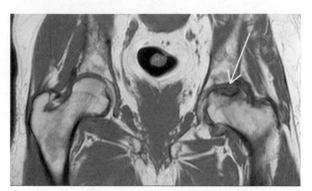

FIGURE 3. **Avascular Necrosis of the Femoral Heads.** Coronal T1W image shows a serpiginous hypointense line along the superior aspect of the left femoral head with loss of normal marrow signal consistent with avascular necrosis.

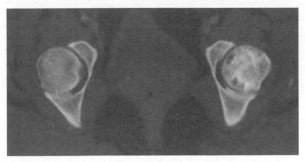

FIGURE 4. **Avascular Necrosis of the Femoral Heads.** Axial CT shows serpiginous band of sclerosis in the left femoral head with associated lucenies as a result of avascular necrosis.

Femoral Neck Fracture

Description: Fractures of the femur are grouped to include the femoral head, femoral neck, intertrochanteric region, femoral shaft, and femoral condyles. Fractures of the femoral neck are divided into three basic types: (1) subcapital (most common); (2) midcervical; and (3) basicervical. The subcapital type is categorized into four stages. The midcervical and basicervical types are rare. The more proximal the fracture line and the more displaced the fracture, the higher the risk for AVN and nonunion.

Etiology: Usually occurs when an elderly person falls.

Epidemiology: Fractures of the femoral neck usually are the result of low-velocity injuries (fall) in the elderly population. About 250,000 subcapital type fractures occur annually in the United States.

Signs and Symptoms: Pain and loss of movement.

Imaging Characteristics:

CT
- Multiplanar reformatted (MPR) images are helpful.
- Helpful if patient has a contraindication to MRI.

MRI
- Fracture appears with low signal on coronal T1-weighted images.
- Fracture line appears with increased signal (hemorrhage and edema) on coronal T2-weighted and STIR images.
- Useful in identifying occult fractures.

Treatment: Depends on the stage, patient's health condition, and surgeon's preference.

Prognosis: Depends on the stage of the fracture. Stage I fractures have the best prognosis.

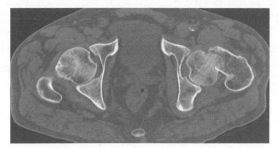

FIGURE 1. **Femoral Neck Fracture.** Axial nonenhanced CT
(NECT) shows a left subcapital femoral neck fracture with
mild impaction posteriorly.

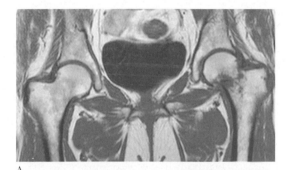

A

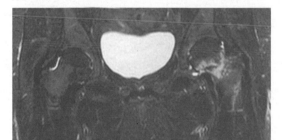

B

FIGURE 2. **Femoral Neck Fracture.** T1W coronal MR (A)
shows an irregular band of low-signal intensity through the
left femoral neck consistent with a fracture. This fracture could
not be seen on the plain radiographs. STIR coronal MR (B) in
the same patient shows high signal in the left femoral neck as a
result of bone marrow edema.

Hip Dislocation

Description: Dislocation of the hip may be associated with a fracture of the acetabulum. The acetabulum or articular socket of the hip is composed of and supported by two columns of bone. The bone of the iliac crest, iliac spines, anterior half of the acetabulum, and the pubis comprise to form the anterior column. The ischium, ischial spine, posterior half of the acetabulum, and the sciatic notch comprise to form the posterior column. The superior portion (i.e., dome or roof) of the acetabulum is the weight-bearing portion of the articular surface that supports the femoral head.

Etiology: Hip dislocations and fractures to the acetabulum or pelvis are commonly caused by trauma.

Epidemiology: Hip dislocations are frequently associated with a femoral fracture. A posterior hip dislocation, the most common type, occurs in approximately 90% of the cases and is frequently associated with a fracture to the posterior margin of the acetabulum.

Signs and Symptoms: Patient presents with pain and loss of function to the extremity affected.

Imaging Characteristics:

CT
- Identify interarticular bony fragments.
- Thin-section multiplanar reconstructed sagittal and coronal images are useful.

MRI
- T1-weighted images appear with low-signal intensity to the affected area.
- T2-weighted images appear with high-signal intensity to the affected area.
- STIR images appear with high-signal intensity to the affected area.
- Useful for the evaluation of avascular necrosis in the head of the femur.

Treatment: Depends on the extent of the injury and other related injuries. Patients will require either an open or closed reduction.

Prognosis: Depends on the extent of the injury and other related injuries.

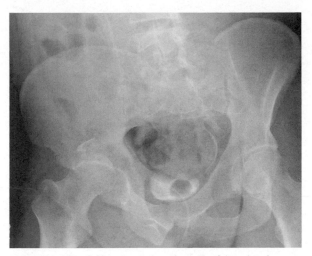

FIGURE 1. **Hip Dislocation.** Judet radiograph of the pelvis shows a fracture of the right acetabulum and posterior dislocation of the right femoral head.

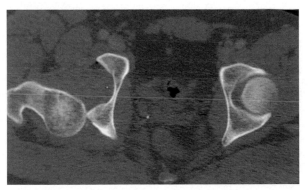

FIGURE 2. **Hip Dislocation.** Axial CT shows the right femoral head dislocated posteriorly out of the acetabulum.

KNEE

Anterior Cruciate Ligament Tear

Description: The anterior cruciate ligament (ACL) is the most commonly injured ligament in the knee. Tearing of the ACL can be classified as complete or partial. Other associated injuries such as O'Donoghue unhappy triad includes, in addition to the tearing of the ACL, tearing of the posterior horn of the medial meniscus and partial tearing of the medial collateral ligament.

Etiology: Injury to the ACL can occur if the knee is (1) externally rotated and abducted with hyperextension, resulting in direct forward displacement of the tibia, or (2) internally rotated with the knee in full extension.

Epidemiology: Injury to the ACL tends to be highly associated with athletic sports (e.g., soccer and basketball) and seems to occur more commonly in females than males.

Signs and Symptoms: Patients usually present with pain and loss of function of the knee.

Imaging Characteristics: MRI is the recommended modality for evaluating the ACL with an accuracy rate of 95% to 100% for complete tears. To better visualize the ACL, the knee should be externally rotated 15° to 20° to align the ligament in the sagittal plane.

MRI

- The normal anterior cruciate ligament is seen as a band of low-signal intensity.
- T2-weighted sagittal images are recommended for the evaluation of the ACL.
- Disruption of the ACL with no normal appearing fibers identified.
- Accuracy of MRI for the ACL is extremely high (95% to 100%).
- There may be associated findings such as joint effusion, meniscal tear, collateral ligament tear, or bone bruise.

Treatment: Complete tearing of the ACL is usually treated surgically. Partial tears are treated symptomatically.

Prognosis: Depends on the severity of the injury and other related injuries to the knee.

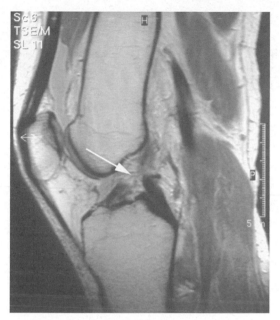

FIGURE 1. **Complete Tear of the Anterior Cruciate Ligament.** T1-weighted sagittal image through the intercondylar notch demonstrates the ACL to be disrupted (*arrow*).

Baker Cyst

Description: A Baker cyst, also known as popliteal cyst, is a distended bursa located in the semimembranous/semitendinous bursa of the popliteal region of the knee.

Etiology: A Baker cyst can be produced by either a herniation of the synovial membrane or leakage of synovial fluid.

Epidemiology: These cysts may result from meniscal injuries, articular cartilage damage, collateral and cruciate ligament injuries, rheumatoid arthritis, loose bodies, and internal derangement of the knee.

Signs and Symptoms: Baker cysts may go unnoticed; however, when they are symptomatic, they manifest with edema and swelling.

Imaging Characteristics:

MRI
- T1-weighted images reveal a hypointense cyst.
- T2-weighted images demonstrate a hyperintense cyst.
- May show associated meniscal tears and joint effusion.

Treatment: May require resection if symptoms persist.

Prognosis: Good.

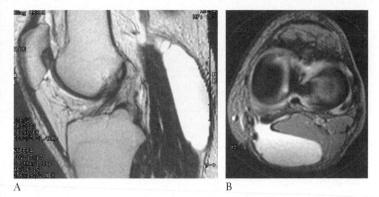

FIGURE 1. Baker Cyst. T2-weighted sagittal (A) and axial (B) MR of the knee demonstrate a large, oval, high-signal mass in the posterior medial aspect of the medial head of the gastrocnemius muscle consistent with a Baker cyst.

Bone Contusion (Bruise)

Description: Bone contusions, also known as bone bruises or microtrabecular fractures, are injuries to the trabecular that occur as a result of an impaction force.

Etiology: Injury to the bony trabeculae usually results from an impaction force.

Epidemiology: Most commonly involve the tibial plateau or the femoral condyles. There is a high incidence of bone bruises in patients with tears to their anterior cruciate ligament.

Signs and Symptoms: Patient presents with pain and a history of an injury.

Imaging Characteristics: Radiographs are usually normal. MRI is very sensitive in detecting bony injuries.

MRI
- T1-weighted images show low-signal intensity within the bony area affected.
- Hyperintense signal intensity is seen in the bony area affected on T2-weighted images.
- STIR images show high-signal intensity at the area of injury.
- The location of the bony injury may indicate associated soft-tissue injuries.
- Good for evaluation of associated ligament and meniscal injury.
- Useful for follow-up evaluation, especially in children.

Treatment: Conservative treatment with a delay in returning to normal activity.

Prognosis: Most bone contusions resolve without complications.

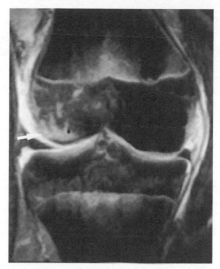

FIGURE 1. Bone Contusion. STIR coronal
MRI shows focal increased signal intensity
(*arrow*) of the medial femoral condyle.

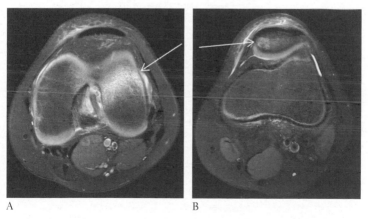

A   B

FIGURE 2. Bone Contusion. Axial proton-density SPIR (spectral presaturation
with inversion recovery) fat-saturation MRI shows increased signal in the lateral
femoral condyle (*arrow*) in (A) and similar increased marrow signal on the medial side
of the patella (B). This pattern of bone bruising is classic for lateral patellar dislocation.

Lateral Collateral Ligament Tear

Description: Is an injury (usually sports related) to the lateral collateral ligament which may result in a tearing of the ligament.

Etiology: Injury results from a force directed at the medial side of the knee, specifically the anteromedial aspect of the tibia.

Epidemiology: Typically occurs in sports which require a lot of quick stops and turns such as soccer, basketball, or as a result of impact sports such as football or hockey.

Signs and Symptoms: Pain is common. Looseness (unstableness) of the knee occurs in more severe cases.

Imaging Characteristics:

MRI
- Useful in evaluating ligament and meniscal tears.
- Better in evaluating complete tears than partial tears.

Treatment: Rest, ice, compression, and nonweight bearing restriction for minor injury. Surgery is recommended for more severe injuries.

Prognosis: Early treatment intervention produces better results.

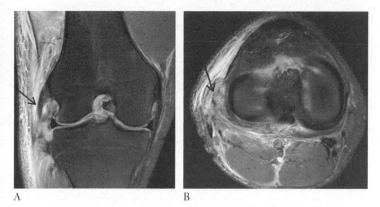

A   B

FIGURE 1. **Lateral Collateral Ligament Tear.** Coronal (A) and axial (B) proton-density SPIR (spectral presaturation with inversion recovery) fat-saturation MRI images show disruption of the lateral collateral ligament with surrounding edema.

Meniscal Tear

Description: A meniscal tear is an injury resulting in a tearing of the crescent-shaped fibrocartilage (meniscus) of the knee joint.

Etiology: Tearing of the menisci may result from acute trauma, repetitive trauma, and progressive degeneration.

Epidemiology: Meniscal tears usually occur as a result of athletic-related injuries. Nonathletic injuries, however, can occur in the aging population. Medial meniscal tears are more common than lateral meniscal tears. Meniscal tears can be associated with anterior cruciate ligament and medial collateral ligament tears, also known as the terrible triad or O'Donoghue sign.

Signs and Symptoms: Pain and discomfort in mobility accompany meniscal tears.

Imaging Characteristics:

MRI
- T1-weighted or proton-density weighted images are the most sensitive for diagnosis of meniscal tear.
- Normal meniscus appears as a low signal.
- Meniscal tear appears as a high signal.
- Meniscal tears may be longitudinal (traumatic) or horizontal (degenerative).
- Meniscal tear may be associated with an anterior cruciate ligament tear, medial collateral ligament tear, joint effusion, or Baker cyst.

Treatment: Depending on the extent of the injury, treatment may vary from physical therapy to meniscectomy.

Prognosis: Varies depending on the extent of injury and other related factors such as age. The patient is encouraged to make a gradual recovery.

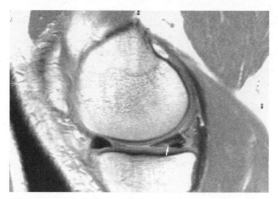

FIGURE 1. Medial Meniscal Tear. Proton-density sagittal image of the knee demonstrates a horizontal tear (*arrow*) of the posterior horn of the medial meniscus that extends to the undersurface.

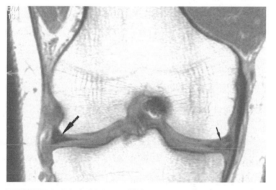

FIGURE 2. Medial Meniscal Tear. Proton-density coronal image of the knee shows a complex tear (*thin arrow*) of the posterior horn of the medial meniscus compared with a normal (*thick arrow*) homogenous low-signal intensity of the lateral meniscus.

Osteoarthritis

Description: Osteoarthritis (OA), commonly referred to as degenerative joint disease or degenerative arthritis, is the result of mechanical or biological events which lead to the deterioration of the articular cartilage.

Etiology: Osteoarthritis may be grouped into primary or secondary types. Primary OA development is unknown. Secondary OA can develop from several different factors such as a fracture into a joint.

Epidemiology: OA is one of the leading causes of work-related disability. Primary OA most commonly affects the hand, wrist, shoulder, hip, knee, foot, and spine. OA affects males and females equally, with frequency increasing with age.

Signs and Symptoms: Pain with weight bearing, limited range of motion, stiffness, and subluxation.

Imaging Characteristics: Diagnostic x-rays useful for initial evaluation, but not as sensitive as MRI.

MRI
- More efficient in detecting early abnormalities involving the articular cartilage.
- Fat-suppressed, three-dimensional, spoiled gradient-echo sequence good for evaluating articular cartilage.

Treatment: Nonsteroidal anti-inflammatory drugs (NSAIDs) commonly used for pain. Weight loss may be helpful. Nutritional supplements such as glucosamine sulfate and chondroitin sulfate have been reported to provide a cure. Various surgical interventions are available.

Prognosis: Better for the primary type of OA. For the secondary type of OA, prognosis depends on the causative factor and other general health-related issues.

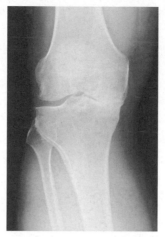

FIGURE 1. Osteoarthritis. AP radiograph of the knee shows severe joint space narrowing of the medial compartment with subchondral sclerosis and marginal osteophyte formation.

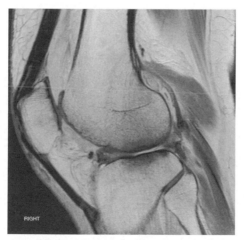

FIGURE 2. Osteoarthritis. Sagittal PD shows joint space narrowing with loss of articular cartilage and loss of normal marrow signal in the subchondral bone as the result of sclerosis.

Osteosarcoma

Description: An osteosarcoma is the most malignant primary bone tumor.

Etiology: In general, there is no known cause. However, radiation has been found to be a predisposing factor associated with the development of bone cancer. Genetic involvement has been linked to patients with retinoblastoma.

Epidemiology: Primary bone cancers are rare, affecting approximately 1 in 100,000 persons. About 4000 to 5000 cases are reported annually. These bone tumors are commonly located in the area of the knee, distal femur, or the proximal tibia. This cancer is generally seen in the younger population, ranging from the early teens to early twenties. Males are more commonly affected than females.

Signs and Symptoms: Patients present with pain, maybe a lump, or both. Approximately 10% of the patients who seek medical attention have already developed metastasis at the time of their initial evaluation. There is a great tendency for osteosarcomas to metastasize to the lungs.

Imaging Characteristics: Plain x-rays are very useful and should be done first. CT is good for the evaluation of bone. MRI is excellent for soft-tissue evaluation.

CT
- Demonstrates bony destruction of the affected area.

MRI
- T1-weighted images show tumor as low-signal intensity.
- T2-weighted images appear as high-signal intensity.
- Disruption of the cortex.
- Associated soft-tissue mass.
- MR is the imaging modality of choice for the evaluation of the extent of the tumor.

Treatment: Surgical resection followed with chemotherapy.

Prognosis: Depends on the staging, if the cancer has spread to other parts of the body (i.e., lung or bone).

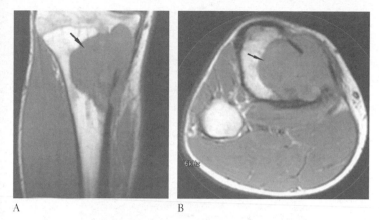

A   B

FIGURE 1. Osteosarcoma. T1-weighted coronal (A) and axial (B) MRIs show large, low-signal-intensity mass (*arrow*) involving the medial aspect of the proximal tibia. There is disruption of the cortex with extension of the tumor medially.

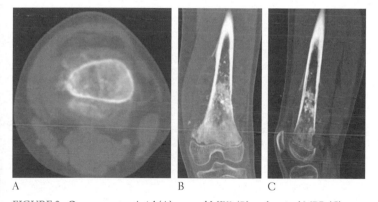

A   B   C

FIGURE 2. Osteosarcoma. Axial (A), coronal MPR (B), and sagittal MPR (C) NECTs of the femur show an aggressive lesion in the distal femur which extends into the soft tissues with cortical breakthrough and osteoid tumor matrix consistent with an osteosarcoma. Note the radially oriented periosteal reaction.

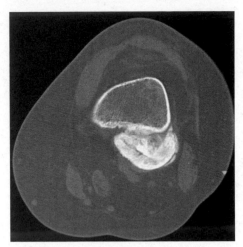

FIGURE 3. **Parosteal Osteosarcoma.** Axial NECT shows a large mass with very dense matrix arising from the posterior surface of the distal femur.

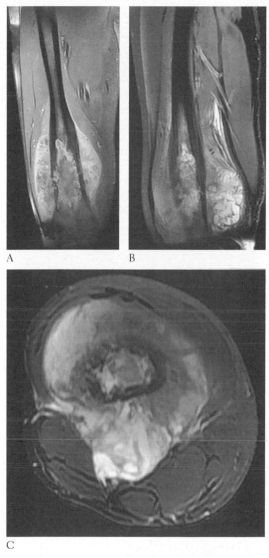

A

B

C

FIGURE 4. **Osteosarcoma.** Coronal T1W FS postcontrast (A), sagittal PD FS (B), and axial T2W FS (C) images show a large-, aggressive-appearing mass in the distal femur with mineralization seen as low signal within the tumor.

Patellar Fracture

Description: Fracture of the patella.

Etiology: Result from either direct or indirect trauma to the knee.

Epidemiology: This fracture represents about 1% of all skeletal fractures. About 60% of patella fractures are classified as transverse. Rare in young children since their skeletal development has not matured.

Signs and Symptoms: Pain and tenderness with associated hemarthrosis.

Imaging Characteristics:

CT
- MPRs good to show fracture.

MRI
- Good to evaluate quadriceps and patella tendon tear.

Treatment: Immobilize the knee for minor injuries. Surgical intervention needed for more advanced cases.

Prognosis: Good.

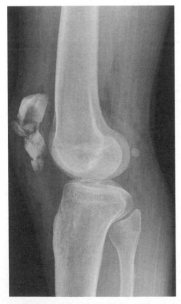

FIGURE 1. **Patellar Fracture.** Lateral radiograph of the knee shows a comminuted patellar fracture.

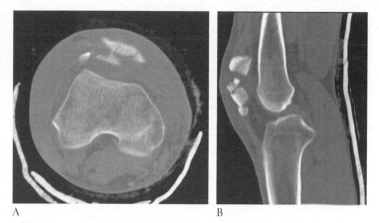

A   B

FIGURE 2. **Patellar Fracture.** Axial (A) and sagittal (B) NECTs of the knee show comminution of the patella in the same patient.

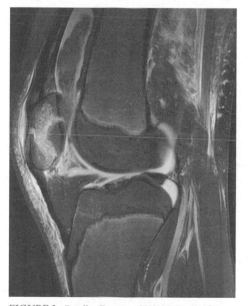

FIGURE 3. **Patellar Fracture.** T2W FS sagittal image of the knee shows disruption of the patellar cortex and high-intensity signal along the fracture plane in a different patient.

Posterior Cruciate Ligament Tear

Description: The posterior cruciate ligament (PCL) may appear with injuries categorized as consisting of ligamentous edema or hemorrhage, partial tearing, or complete tearing of the ligament.

Etiology: Tearing of the posterior cruciate ligament occurs as the result of a posterior force directed to the flexed knee or forced hyperextension.

Epidemiology: Tearing of the PCL occurs frequently in patients diagnosed with dislocation of the knee. Posterior cruciate ligament tears are not as common as anterior cruciate ligament tears.

Signs and Symptoms: Injuries to the knee involving tearing of the posterior cruciate ligament present with pain, loss of motion or disability, and the possibility of vascular and neurologic complications.

Imaging Characteristics:

MRI
- T1- and T2-weighted images demonstrate the normal PCL as a low-signal structure.
- T1-weighted images show poorly defined PCL.
- In acute tears, fluid and edema appear bright (hyperintense) with a high signal on T2-weighted pulse sequences.

Treatment: Depending on the severity of the injury, surgical intervention may be performed when there has been a tearing of the posterior cruciate ligament.

Prognosis: Depending on the degree of injury and other factors such as method of treatment and the patient's history, the patient's recovery and outcome may vary.

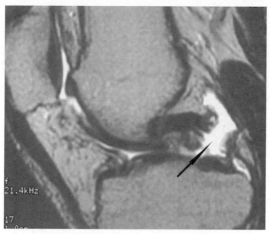

FIGURE 1. Tear of the Posterior Cruciate Ligament.
T2-weighted sagittal image of the knee demonstrates a defect
in the posterior cruciate ligament. There is high-signal intensity
fluid collection at the site of the tear (*arrow*).

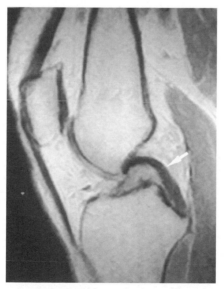

**FIGURE 2. Tear of the Posterior Cruciate
Ligament.** T1-weighted image of a normal
posterior cruciate ligament (*arrow*).

Quadriceps Tear

Description: A tearing or rupturing of the tendon of the quadriceps muscle usually occurs transversely and at the osteotendinous junction.

Etiology: Usually occurs as a result of forced muscle contraction or trauma.

Epidemiology: These injuries occur in the young athlete with either forced muscle contraction or direct trauma or in the elderly through a degenerative area.

Signs and Symptoms: Patient presents with pain at the site of the injury.

Imaging Characteristics: MRI is the imaging modality of choice.

MRI
- MRI is helpful in determining if the tear is partial or complete.
- Disruption or discontinuity of the quadriceps tendon.
- Increased signal intensity of the muscle/tendon on T2-weighted images.

Treatment: Surgical repair is required as soon as possible.

Prognosis: In general, the results are good.

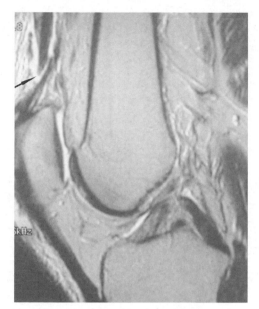

FIGURE 1. **Quadriceps Tear.** T2-weighted sagittal MR image shows disruption (*arrow*) with area of increased signal intensity in projection of the quadriceps tendon.

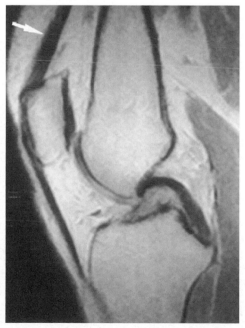

FIGURE 2. **Quadriceps Tear.** Normal quadriceps tendon (*arrow*).

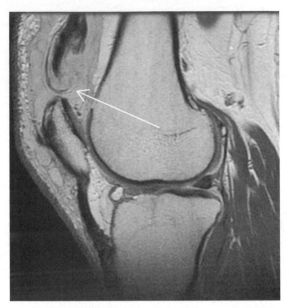

FIGURE 3. **Quadriceps Tear.** Sagittal PD fast spin-echo (FSE) image shows disruption of the normally straight, dark quadriceps tendon with surrounding edema.

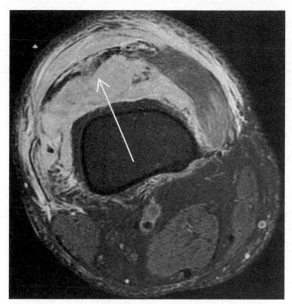

FIGURE 4. **Quadriceps Tear.** Axial PD FSE FS image shows
similar findings (*arrow*) as in Figure 3.

Radiographic Occult Fracture

Description: These are fractures that are difficult to see radiographically, such as stress fractures. These fractures are considered to be occult or equivocal fractures and may be evaluated with MRI. Historically, radio-nuclide bone scans were performed to evaluate these injuries; however, MRI has proven to be cost-effective, efficient, and able to detect these types of bony injuries.

Etiology: These fractures occur as a result of trauma or metabolic disorder.

Epidemiology: Occult fractures can occur at any age. Stress fractures in children and adults are associated with athletic activities; in the elderly, they can occur as a result of a metabolic disorder.

Signs and Symptoms: Patient presents with pain in the area of the injury.

Imaging Characteristics:

MRI
- T1-weighted images show the fracture as low-signal intensity.
- STIR images show the edema and hemorrhage associated with the fracture line as a high-signal intensity.

Treatment: Depends on the type and location of the fracture.

Prognosis: Generally good with early diagnosis and treatment. Avascular necrosis of the femoral head is a complication of the femur near the fracture.

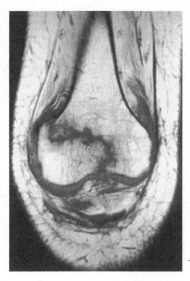

FIGURE 1. Fracture of the Medial Femoral Condyle. T1-weighted coronal MR image of the knee shows oblique fracture (low signal) of the medial femoral condyle extending to the articular margin or joint space. Note: Plain x-rays of the knee were negative.

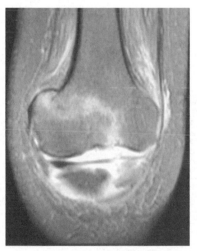

FIGURE 2. Fracture of the Medial Femoral Condyle. STIR coronal MR image of the knee (same patient as in Figure 1) shows an oblique fracture of the medial femoral condyle as high signal.

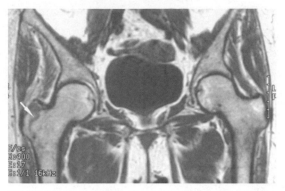

FIGURE 3. Fracture of the Greater Trochanter. T1-weighted coronal MRI of the pelvis shows a fracture of the greater trochanter of the right femur (*arrow*). Note: Plain x-rays of the hip were negative.

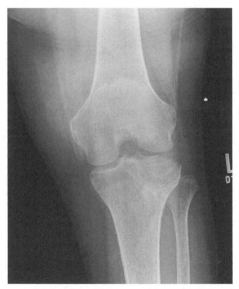

FIGURE 4. Fracture of the Medial Femoral Condyle. No fracture is clearly seen on the AP knee radiograph.

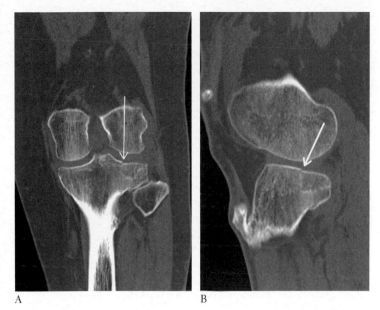

A   B

FIGURE 5. **Fracture of the Medial Femoral Condyle.** Coronal (A) and sagittal (B) MPR NECTs of the knee show a minimally depressed lateral tibial plateau fracture (*arrows*). Compare with Figure 4.

Tibial Plateau Fracture

Description: A tibial plateau fracture is an intra-articular fracture which typically produces large hemarthrose (blood in the joint) in the joint.

Etiology: This type of fracture usually results from a valgus load with impaction at the lateral tibial condyle.

Epidemiology: Approximately 80% of these fractures affect the lateral tibial plateau.

Signs and Symptoms: Patient presents with pain and loss of function.

Imaging Characteristics:

CT
- MPRs are helpful in showing bony fragments and degree of displacement.

MRI
- Good to evaluate menisci, cruciate, and collateral ligaments.

Treatment: Surgery.

Prognosis: A valgus angular deformity may be seen when compared to the opposite tibia.

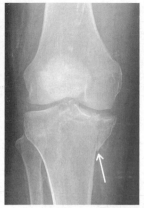

FIGURE 1. **Tibial Plateau Fracture.** AP radiograph of the knee shows a comminuted minimally displaced medial tibial plateau fracture.

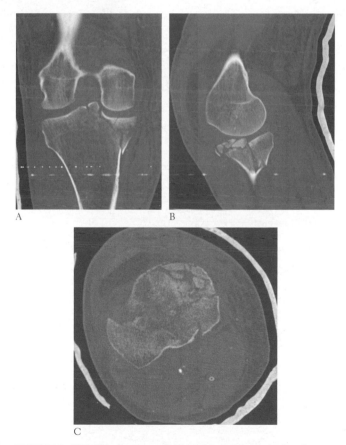

FIGURE 2. **Tibial Plateau Fracture.** This is better characterized on the coronal MPR (A), sagittal MPR (B), and axial (C) images of the knee.

Unicameral (Simple) Bone Cyst

Description: Unicameral bone cyst, or sometimes referred to as simple bone cyst, is a fluid-filled cyst. This bone cyst may present as a single-chambered cyst, or with a bubbly, multichambered appearance.

Etiology: The cause of these benign lesions is still unknown.

Epidemiology: Unicameral bone cysts represent approximately 3% to 5% of the primary bone tumors. Though unicameral bone cysts typically present in the first two decades of life, about 80% of these cases commonly occur between the ages of 3 and 14 years. In approximately 90% of the cases, these bone cysts affect the proximal humerus, proximal femur, and proximal tibia. There is a male predominance of 3:1.

Signs and Symptoms: This bony lesion is typically asymptomatic unless fractured. Approximately two-thirds of the patients present with a pathologic fracture. Pain and loss of function accompany a fracture.

Imaging Characteristics: Plain x-rays are usually diagnostic. MRI should always be correlated with plain films.

CT
- The fluid-filled cyst appears hypodense.

MRI
- This fluid-filled cyst is seen as a homogeneous low-signal intensity on a T1-weighted image.
- T2-weighted images demonstrate high-signal intensity.

Treatment: Surgical intervention is the treatment of choice.

Prognosis: Good; this is a benign tumor, with a small chance of recurrence.

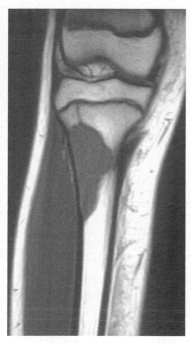

FIGURE 1. **Unicameral Bone Cyst.**
T1-weighted coronal MRI shows low-signal-intensity lesion involving the proximal tibia.

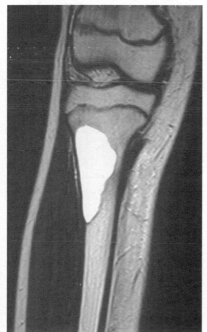

FIGURE 2. **Unicameral Bone Cyst.**
T2-weighted MRI shows well-defined high-signal-intensity mass of the proximal tibia. The cortex is intact and there is no associated soft-tissue mass.

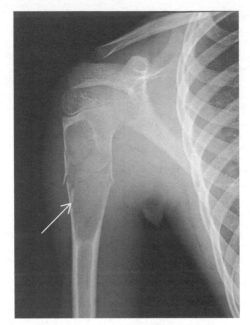

FIGURE 3. **Unicameral Bone Cyst.** Radiograph of the right shoulder shows a large, sharply defined lucency in the proximal humerus with a pathologic fracture and "fallen fragment" sign (*arrow*).

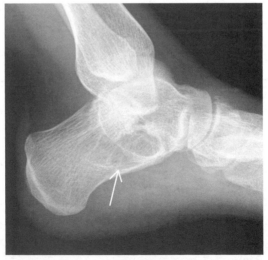

FIGURE 4. **Unicameral Bone Cyst.** Lateral radiograph of the calcaneus shows a well-marginated lucency.

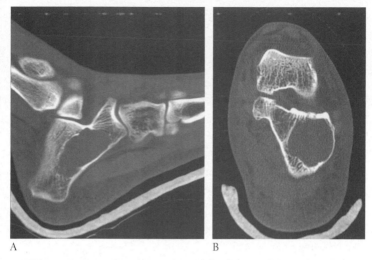

A   B

FIGURE 5. **Unicameral Bone Cyst.** Sagittal (A) and coronal (B) CTs show fluid density with this area and no internal matrix.

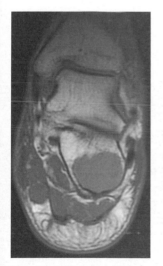

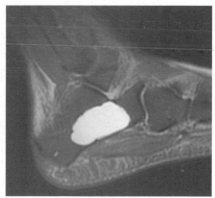

FIGURE 6. **Unicameral Bone Cyst.** T1W coronal image shows intermediate signal within the lesion.

FIGURE 7. **Unicameral Bone Cyst.** Sagittal PD FS image shows uniform high-intensity-fluid signal within this simple bone cyst.

ANKLE AND FEET

Achilles Tendon Tear

Description: The Achilles tendon is the longest and strongest tendon in the foot and ankle. Tearing of the Achilles tendon may be classified as either partial or complete.

Etiology: Tearing of the Achilles tendon usually results from indirect trauma such as athletic or strenuous activities.

Epidemiology: Athletic-related injuries can result at any age. Injuries associated with strenuous activities are most common between 30 and 50 years of age. Achilles tendon tears occur more commonly in males than females.

Signs and Symptoms: Patients usually present with pain, local swelling, and an inability to raise their toes on the affected side.

Imaging Characteristics: MRI is the useful modality for the detection of an Achilles tendon tear.

MRI

- MRI is accurate in demonstrating partial and complete tears and following the progress of healing.
- Partial tear shows increased signal intensity within the tendon on T2-weighted images.
- Complete tear shows as a wavy and lax tendon or discontinuity, retraction, and fraying of the ends. Increased signal at the site of the tear.
- T2-weighted double-echo sagittal and axial images are the most useful.

Treatment: Partial tearing of the Achilles tendon may not require surgical intervention. Instead, immobilization and reduced weight bearing may be more appropriate. Patients with complete tears need surgical intervention.

Prognosis: The patient's outcome may vary depending on the extent of injury and method of treatment. Other factors to consider include the patient's age and mobility.

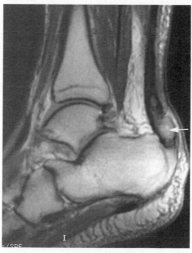

FIGURE 1. Achilles Tendon Tear.
T1-weighted sagittal MR of the ankle
demonstrates thickening and intrasubstance
increased signal (*arrow*) within the distal
Achilles tendon, consistent with a chronic
tear.

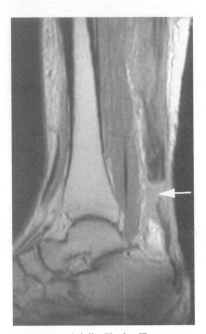

FIGURE 2. Achilles Tendon Tear.
T1-weighted sagittal MR of the ankle
demonstrates a complete acute tear
(*arrow*) of the Achilles tendon near the
musculotendinous junction.

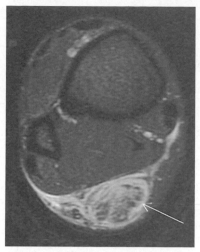

FIGURE 3. Achilles Tendon Tear. Axial T2W FS image shows an enlarged, ill-defined Achilles tendon with increased signal consistent with a tear (*arrow*).

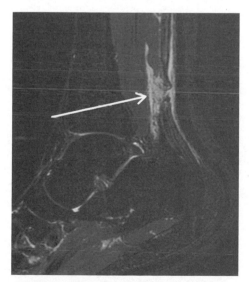

FIGURE 4. Achilles Tendon Tear. Sagittal STIR image clearly shows disruption of the Achilles tendon and surrounding high-signal edema.

Brodie Abscess

Description: A localized form of subacute osteomyelitis which occurs most often in the metaphysis of long bones in children.

Etiology: The pathogen usually responsible is *Staphylococcus aureus*.

Epidemiology: The lower extremities, especially the tibia, are more commonly affected than the upper extremities. Males are slightly more affected than females. Common age for occurrence is between 2 and 15 years.

Signs and Symptoms: Symptoms are typically mild with persistent local pain.

Imaging Characteristics:

CT
- IV postcontrast shows abscess with rim enhancement.

MRI
- Fat-suppressed T2-weighted images show high-signal intense abscess.
- Postgadolinium images show abscess with rim enhancement.

Treatment: Biopsy and curettage are required for diagnosis. Antibiotics are usually given.

Prognosis: Full recovery is expected.

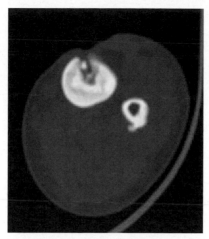

FIGURE 1. Brodie Abscess. Noncontrast CT of the left leg shows an area of bone destruction within the anterior tibia surrounded by increased sclerosis.

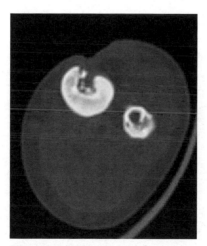

FIGURE 2. Brodie Abscess. Bone sequestrum within the abscess.

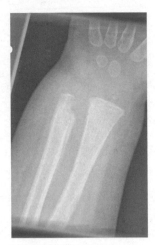

FIGURE 3. Brodie Abscess.
Plain radiograph of the
wrist shows irregularity and
destruction of the bone along
the distal ulna with periosteal
reaction and surrounding soft-
tissue swelling.

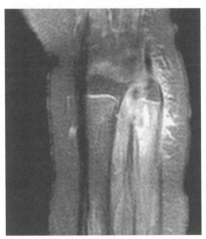

FIGURE 4. Brodie Abscess. Coronal
T1W contrasted MR of the wrist shows rim
enhancement of the distal ulna with an area of
bone destruction.

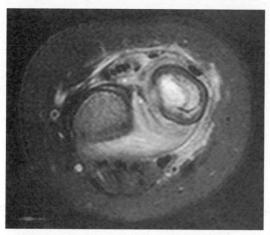

FIGURE 5. Brodie Abscess. Axial T2W SPIR MR image showing increased signal intensity in the distal ulna and surrounding edema.

Diabetic Foot

Description: Infection and ulceration in the foot of a diabetic patient.

Etiology: Peripheral neuropathy affects sensory, motor, and autonomic nerve pathways which desensitize the patient to early warning signs of pain or pressure from footwear. Vascular disease is the second risk factor associated with developing ulcer and infection in the diabetic foot. The third risk factor is a decline in a diabetic patient's immune system.

Epidemiology: About 15% of individuals with diabetes will have a foot ulcer in their lifetime. About 85% of nontraumatic lower extremity amputations (LEA) occur as a result of diabetic foot ulcers. Patients who have had a foot ulcer are at risk of an LEA by a factor of 8.

Signs and Symptoms: Early symptoms may include persistent pain, redness, localized warmth, and swelling of the affected foot.

Imaging Characteristics:

MRI

- MRI sensitive to bony involvement of osteomyelitis.
- Osteomyelitis: T1W shows decreased signal in focal bone marrow; T2W shows increased signal in focal bone marrow; and T1W with gadolinium shows focal enhancement with or without cortical destruction.
- Cellulitis: Fat-saturated T2W shows increased signal in bone marrow; and T1W with gadolinium shows absence of bone changes.
- Abscess: Fat-saturated T2W shows well-defined high-signal collection in soft tissue; and T1W with gadolinium may or may not show rim enhancement.
- STIR shows osteomyelitis as hyperintense.

Treatment: Preventive strategies are the primary focus in reducing the chances of developing a foot ulcer. If a foot ulcer develops, management of systemic diabetes and debridement of any necrotic tissue is usually performed. Vascular surgery consultation may be required to evaluate possible amputation.

Prognosis: Poor.

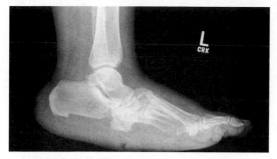

FIGURE 1. **Diabetic Foot.** Lateral plain radiograph of a diabetic foot with air in the plantar soft tissues with surrounding edema consistent with an ulcer.

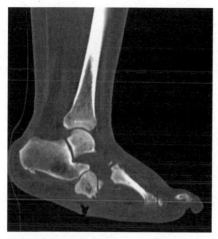

FIGURE 2. **Diabetic Foot.** Noncontrast sagittal CT of the same patient confirms subcutaneous gas and underlying bone destruction consistent with osteomyelitis.

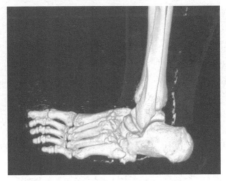

FIGURE 3. **Multiple Tarsal-Metatarsal Joint Dislocations.** 3D volume rendered image of the same patient shows extensive neuropathic joint changes consistent with Charcot foot.

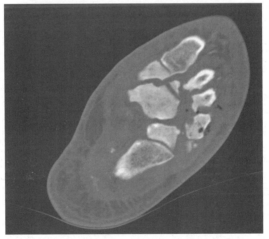

FIGURE 4. **Diabetic Foot.** Axial NECT showing low-attenuation subcutaneous air, bone destruction, and edema consistent with gangrene and osteomyelitis.

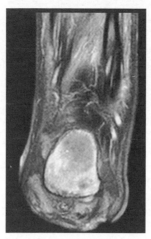

FIGURE 5. Diabetic Foot. T2W coronal MR of the foot shows an ulcer of the skin overlying the calcaneus and increased signal within the subcutaneous tissues and calcaneus. This is consistent with osteomyelitis.

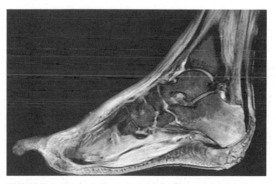

FIGURE 6. Diabetic Foot. Proton-density sagittal shows increased signal in the calcaneus and overlying tissues, with a posterior skin ulcer. This is consistent with osteomyelitis.

Peroneal Tendon Tear

Description: A tear of a peroneal tendon. There are two peroneal tendons (peroneus brevis and peroneus longus) which are positioned along the lateral side of the ankle posterior to the lateral malleolus. Of the two peroneal tendons, the peroneus brevis is more commonly affected.

Etiology: Most common trauma is a lateral ankle sprain. Subluxations and dislocations may also cause injury.

Epidemiology: Following the Achilles tendon and the posterior tibial tendon, the peroneal tendons are the third most commonly injured tendons at the ankle. The peroneus brevis is more commonly affected with tendinopathy and is associated with a tear known as split peroneus brevis syndrome, which is a longitudinal tearing of this tendon. With this condition, the peroneus brevis is impinged between the peroneus longus and the tibia.

Signs and Symptoms: Patients present with pain and swelling over the lateral malleolus.

Imaging Characteristics:

CT
- Helpful in detecting avulsion fractures of the lateral malleolus.

MRI
- Increased internal tendon signal on T1- and T2-weighted images most common for tear.
- Axial and sagittal planes show peroneal tendons proximal to the base of the fifth metatarsal.
- T2-weighted and T2*-weighted gradient echo are helpful in detecting subluxations and dislocations.

Treatment: Nonsteroidal anti-inflammatory drugs (NASIDs) are helpful in reducing pain and inflammation. Conservative therapy may include immobilization and corticosteroid injection. Partial or complete tendon tear will probably require surgery.

Prognosis: Good recovery is expected.

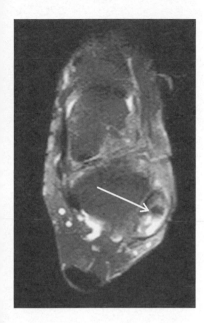

FIGURE 1. Peroneal Tendon Tear. Axial T2W FS image of the ankle shows hyperintense signal within the peroneus brevis tendon and sheath (*arrow*).

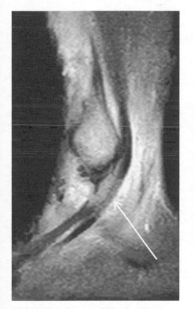

FIGURE 2. Peroneal Tendon Tear. Sagittal PD FSE FS image shows increased signal in the peroneus brevis tendon and surrounding soft tissues due to edema.

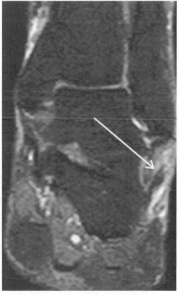

FIGURE 3. Peroneal Tendon Tear. Coronal IR shows similar findings as in Figure 2.

Sinus Tarsi Syndrome

Description: Sinus tarsi syndrome is associated with a posttraumatic lateral hindfoot pain and instability.

Etiology: Inversion-related injuries to the ankle.

Epidemiology: Trauma (inversion) related in about 70% to 80% of cases may have lateral tendon tears with possible damaged nerves. Inflammatory arthropathies are associated with the remaining 30%.

Signs and Symptoms: Patient presents with lateral foot pain and feeling of hindfoot instability.

Imaging Characteristics:

MRI
- May not be able to see the sinus tarsi fat; however, this may not indicate sinus tarsi syndrome.
- Low signal on T1-weighted images.
- High (inflammatory) signal or low (fibrotic) signal on T2-weighted images.

Treatment: Steroid injection, surgical reconstruction of the sinus tarsi ligaments.

Prognosis: Good.

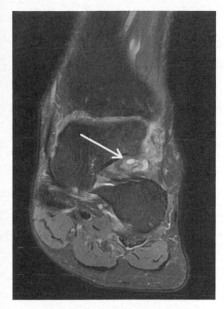

FIGURE 1. **Sinus Tarsi Syndrome.** Coronal IR shows increased fluid signal (edema) surrounding the sinus tarsi ligaments which also have abnormally high signal.

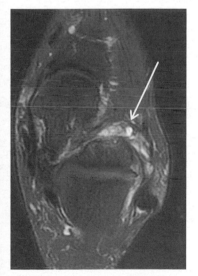

FIGURE 2. **Sinus Tarsi Syndrome.** Axial IR sequence shows similar findings, as shown in Figure 1.

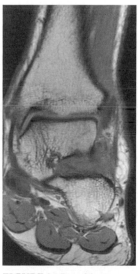

FIGURE 3. **Sinus Tarsi Syndrome.** T1W coronal image shows loss of the normal, high-intensity sinus tarsi fat signal which has been replaced with intermediate fluid signal.

VASCULAR

Peripheral Arterial Disease

Description: Peripheral arterial disease (PAD) is a vascular condition that occurs when the blood supply to internal organs, arms, and legs (extremities) becomes partially or completely blocked, usually as a result of atherosclerosis plaque.

Etiology: Most commonly occurs as a result of atherosclerosis. Genetic and lifestyle factors also contribute to plaque development.

Epidemiology: African Americans are at greater risk than Caucasians. Approximately 5% of 50-year-old people are affected.

Signs and Symptoms: Asymptomatic in many patients. Intermittent claudication (limping or lameness) type symptoms may cause leg pain and cramping during physical activities such as walking or climbing stairs. A weak or absent pulse in the legs or feet, slow healing of sores on the toes, feet, or legs, pale or bluish skin color, lower temperature in one leg compared to the other leg, and erectile dysfunction in men are additional symptoms.

Imaging Characteristics: Doppler ultrasound including ankle brachial index (ABI) is best for initial screening.

CT
- CT Angiography (CTA) from the level of the renal arteries (T12 vertebra) to the feet is good for showing stenosis, occlusion, thrombus, embolus, and aneurysms affecting the peripheral arteries.
- Curved plane reformations (CPRs), maximum intensity projections (MIPs), and volume renderings (VRs) are good to assist with evaluating angiographic maps of the arterial tree.

MRI
- MR angiography (MRA) from the level of the renal arteries (T12 vertebra) to the feet is good for showing stenosis, occlusion, thrombus, embolus, and aneurysms affecting the peripheral arteries.

Treatment: May range from a variety of medications for lowering cholesterol and high blood pressure, controlling blood sugar, blood clot prevention, to thrombolytic therapy, angioplasty, or bypass surgery. Lifestyle changes such as dietary and regular exercise may be prescribed.

Prognosis: Prevention by maintaining a healthy lifestyle is best.

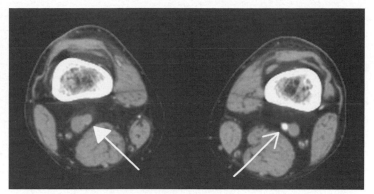

FIGURE 1. Peripheral Arterial Disease. Axial CECT shows no filling of the right popliteal artery (*closed arrow*) compared to the normal-appearing high-attenuation artery on the left (*open arrow*).

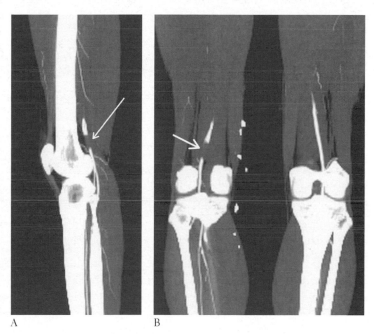

A   B

FIGURE 2. Peripheral Arterial Disease. Sagittal (A) and coronal (B) MIP CTA images of the legs show a filling defect in the popliteal artery due to occlusive thrombus.

MISCELLANEOUS

Ewing Sarcoma

Description: Ewing sarcoma is a highly malignant type of bone cancer primarily found in children. Commonly found in the pelvis and long bones (75%), it may also be seen in the shoulder girdle, ribs, and vertebral body.

Etiology: Unknown; however, there is some information to support that certain changes in a cell's DNA may cause the cell to become cancerous.

Epidemiology: This is the most common type of bone cancer affecting children younger than 10 years. Males more commonly with a male-to-female ration of 2:1. About 90% to 95% of cases occur between the ages of 5 and 25 years, with the majority occurring between 5 and 14 years. About 96% of all cases affect Caucasians.

Signs and Symptoms: Pain is usually experienced. Some may experience fever, erythema, and swelling which is suggestive of osteomyelitis.

Imaging Characteristics: A nuclear medicine bone scan is recommended to evaluate bone since this is the second most common site of metastases. X-ray shows an osteolytic process in the diaphysis of a long bone.

CT
- Useful to evaluate the chest since the lungs are the most common site of metastases.

MRI
- Better than CT for staging.
- T1-weighted images appear with hypointense to isointense to muscle.
- T2-weighted images appear with high signal.

Treatment: Ewing sarcoma is very radiosensitive. Decision between radiation and surgery for amputation is made on an individual case-by-case basis. Neoadjuvant chemotherapy (i.e., chemotherapy is given prior to cancer surgery or radiotherapy) may also be considered to reduce the size of the cancer and increase the chance of success.

Prognosis: The overall 5-year survival rate has improved to about 70% to 75%. If metastases are present, the 5-year survival rate is about 20% to 30%.

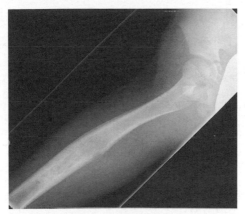

FIGURE 1. Ewing Sarcoma. Lateral radiograph of the right femur shows an ill-defined permeative destructive lesion in the mid-diaphysis with an "onion skin" type of periosteal reaction.

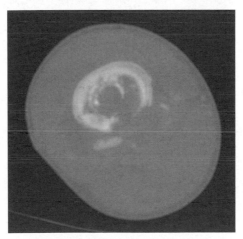

FIGURE 2. Ewing Sarcoma. Axial NECT shows an intramedullary mass resulting in bone destruction and an aggressive periosteal reaction.

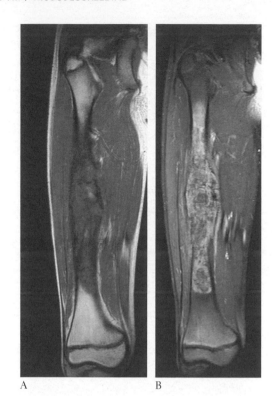

A   B

FIGURE 3. **Ewing Sarcoma.** Coronal T1W without
gadolinium (A) MR of the femur shows a low-signal-
intensity, expansile mass in the mid-diaphysis. Image (B) is
a coronal T1W gadolinium-enhanced image and appears
bright.

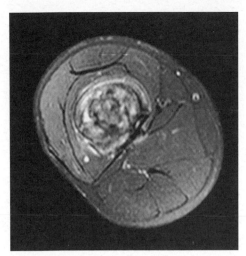

FIGURE 4. **Ewing Sarcoma.** Axial T2W shows increased signal intensity within the mass.

INDEX